TRACKING OUTPATIENTS

USING THE E-HEALTH SYSTEM TO ENSURE POSITIVE TREATMENT PROGRESS FOR HOSPITAL SERVICES' EFFECTIVENESS FOR CLIENT TRACKING AND COMMUNICATION AT GOLDEN YEARS CARE

DR. TAMER SABRY, BSW, MBA, D.B.A

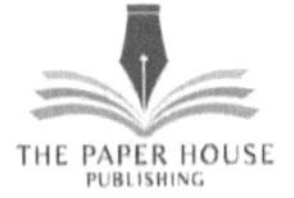

THE PAPER HOUSE
PUBLISHING

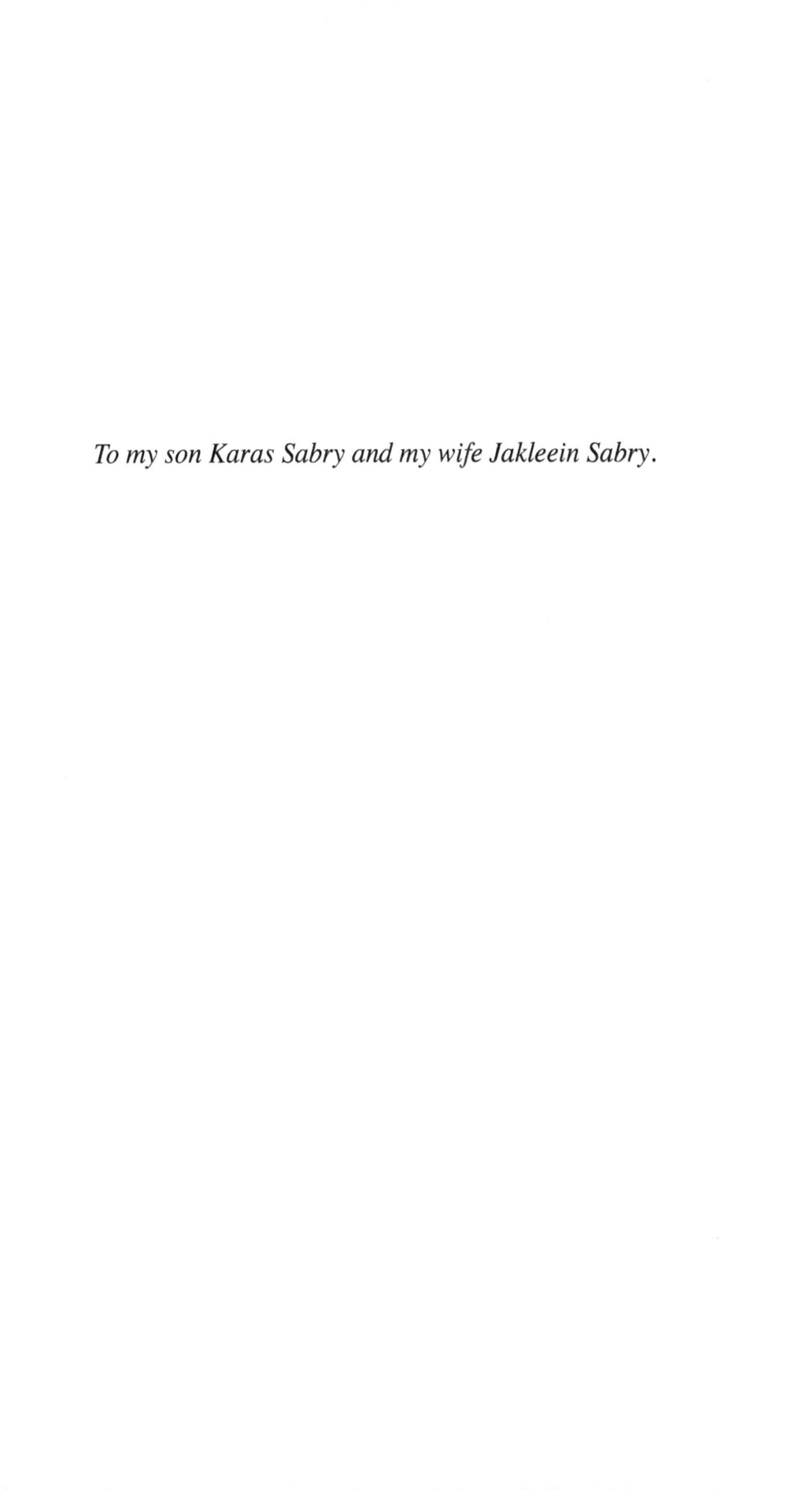

To my son Karas Sabry and my wife Jakleein Sabry.

CONTENTS

ABSTRACT   1
PUBLIC PROFILE & URL   2

SECTION 1: INTRODUCTION TO DOCTORAL
RESEARCH PROJECT   3
Background of the Problem & Problem Statement

PROBLEM STATEMENT   7
Purpose Statement & Significance of the Study
Problem Statement   7
Specific Problem Statement   8
Purpose statement   8
Significance of the Study   9

LITERATURE SUPPORT   13
Advancing Theory
Project Type & Organization Permission   13
Project Type   13
Organization Permission   14
Research Questions and Methodology   14
Research Question   14
Methodology   14
Data Collection   15
Data Analysis   16

SECTION 2: LITERATURE SUPPORT   19
Description of the Problem and Business Practices
Description of the Problem   19
Description of Business Practices   20
Discussion on Previous Research   21
Research Framework   22
Key Tenets of the Technology Acceptance
Model (TAM)   22

Connection to the Study Approach and Research
Questions   23
Relevance to Instrument Development and Data
Analysis   23

COMPLETE LITERATURE REVIEW   29
Introduction   29
Literature Search Strategy   30

THEORETICAL FOUNDATION   33
Theory: The Technology Acceptance Model (TAM)
Theoretical Background   33
Key Concepts and Propositions   33
Literature Analysis   34
The Rationale for Theory Choice   35
Relationship with the Present Study   35

LITERATURE REVIEW   37
Summary   59
The Present Study   60

SECTION 3: RESEARCH METHODOLOGY   63
Role of the Researcher Research Methodology
Discussion on the Population and Sampling   64
Study Population   64
Study Sample   64
Eligible Participants   65
Data Security and Participant Confidentiality   66
Reasons for Eligibility   66
Population Sampling Process   67
Study Samples and Methods for Determining the
Samples   68
Detailed Descriptions   70
Recruiting   70
Selection   70
Procedures for Assigning to Groups   71
Gaining Access to the Sample   71
The Actual Participants   72
Summary   72
Data Collection and Analysis   73

Data Collection 73

Data Analysis 73

Assumptions, Limitations, Delimitations 75

Assumptions 75

Limitations 77

Delimitations 78

SECTION 4: RESULTS, DISCUSSIONS AND IMPLICATIONS 81

Results 81

Underutilization of E-Health Services in Healthcare Practices 81

Employee Resistance to Organizational Change in Healthcare Settings 82

DISCUSSIONS 83

Underutilization of E-Health Services 83

Employee Resistance to Organizational Change 84

Practical Implications for Healthcare Organizations 84

Relationship of Findings 85

Implications and Recommendations for Future Research 87

Implications 87

Recommendations for Future Research 88

Summary and Study Conclusion 92

Summary 92

Conclusion 93

REFERENCES 97

LETTER TO THE FACILITY REQUESTING ACCESS PERMISSION (APPENDIX A) 109

LIST OF INTERVIEW QUESTIONS (APPENDIX B) 111

This research endeavors to uncover the challenges Adult Medical Daycare facilities in the State of New Jersey encounter in establishing effective aftercare follow-up procedures, resulting in untapped opportunities for optimized patient care. This study delves into the complex dynamics of underutilization and resistance to organizational change within this context. The findings illuminate the critical role that comprehensive training and robust support systems play in driving the adoption of E-Health services while simultaneously addressing data privacy and security concerns. Furthermore, this study emphasizes the pivotal impact of employee involvement and the influence of organizational culture in ameliorating resistance to transformative changes. Guided by the Technology Acceptance Model, this investigation examines the intricate interplay between these elements, culminating in actionable recommendations for healthcare institutions. By embracing these insights, healthcare organizations can effectively harness the potential of E-Health services, leading to tangible advancements in patient care delivery and operational efficiency.

TRACKING OUTPATIENTS, USING THE E-HEALTH SYSTEM TO ENSURE POSITIVE TREATMENT PROGRESS FOR HOSPITAL SERVICES' EFFECTIVENESS FOR CLIENT TRACKING AND COMMUNICATION AT GOLDEN YEARS CARE

PUBLIC PROFILE & URL

www.linkedin.com/in/dr-tamer-sabry-bsw-mba-d-b-a-hcml-469971279

Dr. Tamer Sabry, BSW, MBA, D.B.A (HCML)
Adjunct Professor
University of the People.
Pasadena, CA

SECTION 1: INTRODUCTION TO DOCTORAL RESEARCH PROJECT

BACKGROUND OF THE PROBLEM & PROBLEM STATEMENT

The healthcare industry has experienced changes in recent years due to the widespread adoption of electronic health records (EHRs) and the implementation of E-Health systems. These technological advancements have the potential to revolutionize care, improve communication among healthcare providers, and enhance overall organizational efficiency. However, despite their benefits, there is a growing concern about how effective and impactful E-Health systems are in addressing the inability of Adult Medical Daycare in the State of New Jersey to institute aftercare follow-up for patients, resulting in missed opportunities for delivering more effective patient care.

Existing research literature has shed light on the importance of E-Health systems in enhancing care and streamlining healthcare processes. Studies conducted by Johnson et al. (2021) have shown outcomes linked to using E-Health systems, such as improved communication among healthcare providers and increased job satisfaction among nurses due to easily accessible healthcare records. Additionally, the gap in existing literature pertains to E-Health systems' deficient implementation and efficacy within specialized healthcare facilities like Adult Medical Daycare in New Jersey. This void underscores real-world obstacles that hinder system integration, yielding inefficiencies and suboptimal patient outcomes.

Like many healthcare institutions, Golden Years Care has introduced an E-Health system to enhance patient care and operational efficiency. Yet, concerns about the system's impact on care quality and facility effectiveness have emerged, specifically regarding the inability to establish effective aftercare follow-up for patients in the State of New Jersey. Staff and patients have identified issues such as delays in accessing records, difficulties navigating the system, and occasional data entry errors. While existing literature mainly highlights the benefits of E-Health systems, there is a lack of studies specifically addressing the unique challenges faced during implementation and usage at individual healthcare facilities. To enhance patient care, it is vital to explore the effectiveness of the E-Health system within New Jersey's Adult Medical Daycare, focusing on aftercare follow-up barriers.

This study focuses on the Adult Medical Daycare in New Jersey's inability to establish patient aftercare follow-up, leading to missed opportunities for enhanced patient care.

Through a case study at Golden Years Care facility, this study aims to investigate staff experiences with the E-Health system, identifying factors influencing its efficiency and effectiveness within the facility. The study seeks to understand Golden Years Care's difficulties in effectively utilizing the E-Health system. Additionally, it aims to explore strategies for improving its functionality.

The importance of this study goes beyond filling a gap in the existing literature. It has implications for healthcare administrators and policymakers. Healthcare facilities can implement targeted interventions to optimize their systems and enhance organizational effectiveness by understanding the challenges and obstacles faced when using E-Health systems. The findings from this study will be a resource for healthcare organizations looking to fully leverage the potential of E-Health systems and streamline healthcare processes. Moreover, in a changing healthcare landscape, it is crucial to continuously assess and improve the implementation and usage of E-Health systems. The results of this study will contribute to the discussion about integrating digital technology into healthcare, leading the way for future research and advancements in this field.

PROBLEM STATEMENT

PURPOSE STATEMENT & SIGNIFICANCE OF
THE STUDY

PROBLEM STATEMENT

The general problem to be addressed is the inability of some healthcare institutions to institute aftercare follow-up for patients, resulting in missed opportunities to deliver more effective patient care.

Supporting sentences

- There were expectations that patient monitoring by healthcare teams would be easier with the development of E-Health platforms. However, due to user restrictions, various specialists have criticized its effectiveness (Kruse et al., 2018).
- The digitization of medical records and the development of communications networks that enable the exchange of health information have opened up significant opportunities to scale up and digitally enhance patient health monitoring and management (Atasoy et al., 2019). However, the practical deployment of digital health technology is

still complicated, particularly in settings with limited resources.

- The opportunities for digital health initiatives also face significant challenges, such as unreliable digital infrastructure and ineffective patient referral systems, which directly result from inadequate linking between E-Health platforms and hospital information systems (Duggal et al., 2023).

SPECIFIC PROBLEM STATEMENT

The specific problem to be addressed is the inability of Adult Medical Daycare in the State of New Jersey to institute aftercare follow-up for patients, resulting in missed opportunities to deliver more effective patient care.

PURPOSE STATEMENT

This qualitative study aims to investigate the challenges and factors contributing to the inability of an Adult Medical Daycare in New Jersey to establish aftercare follow-up for patients, thereby hindering the delivery of effective patient care. Specifically, the study intends to describe the staff members' experiences and perceptions of using the E-Health system, identify potential causes of inefficiency, and develop insights into enhancing system effectiveness. The utilization of E-Health systems is the dependent variable, whereas the factors that affect the efficacy and inefficiency of the system are the dependent variables.

Covariate variables may include the staff members' roles, years of experience, and familiarity with E-Health technology. Through in-depth interviews and thematic analysis, this research aims to provide valuable data and workable solutions for optimizing the E-Health system, ultimately improving patient care and organizational practices at Golden Years Care facility.

SIGNIFICANCE OF THE STUDY

The Significance of the Study lies in its potential to address the specific problem of the inability of Adult Medical Daycare in the State of New Jersey to establish aftercare follow-up for patients, thus offering insights into enhancing patient care effectiveness. Moreover, the study aims to promote positive social change by providing insights that could improve healthcare service delivery and patient outcomes. The significance of this study is underscored by its potential to address the critical problem of the inability of Adult Medical Daycare in the State of New Jersey to establish effective aftercare follow-up for patients. This issue has far-reaching implications for patient care outcomes and healthcare service delivery, making the study highly important and relevant.

The study's findings can significantly enhance patient care effectiveness within the Adult Medical Daycare. By investigating the factors influencing the establishment of aftercare follow-up, the study can uncover barriers and challenges hindering the provision of comprehensive and continuous patient care. As a result, the insights gained from this study can inform targeted strategies and interventions that enable healthcare practitioners to overcome these barriers and ensure that patients receive the necessary follow-up care (De Grood et al., 2016). Conducting this study also holds broader benefits for the field of healthcare. The insights generated through exploring E-Health system utilization and aftercare follow-up can contribute to the existing knowledge on healthcare service delivery and technology implementation.

The study's outcomes can provide valuable information for leaders and practitioners in healthcare organizations, enabling them to make informed decisions about integrating E-Health systems and enhancing aftercare practices. Furthermore, the study's results can contribute to positive social change by improving patient outcomes and experiences. Effective aftercare follow-up is essential for patients' overall well-being and recovery, and addressing the identified problem can lead to better patient satisfaction and quality of life (Santana et al., 2018). As patients experience improved aftercare and continuity of care, the study's impact on social change extends to the larger community, promoting a healthier population and fostering a positive healthcare environment.

The study's significance is underscored by the imperative need to address the identified problem. In today's rapidly evolving healthcare landscape, where technology plays a pivotal role in patient care, understanding the challenges and barriers to effective aftercare follow-up is crucial. Without a comprehensive exploration of these factors, the Adult Medical Daycare and similar healthcare facilities may continue to miss opportunities for delivering optimal patient care, ultimately impacting patient outcomes and organizational effectiveness.

This study explores the factors affecting the E-Health system's effectiveness at a New Jersey Adult Medical Daycare, particularly in implementing aftercare follow-up for patients, aiming to enhance patient care opportunities. Through qualitative single-case study research and interviews, this study will delve into staff members' perceptions and experiences with the system, which can enrich our understanding of how E-Health systems are utilized in healthcare organizations. The findings may generate new insights into the complex interactions between technology, healthcare professionals, and patient care, potentially leading to refining and expanding existing theories in health informatics and healthcare management.

The study's investigation into nurses' job satisfaction and E-Health system utilization addresses missed opportunities in patient care, contributing to a deeper understanding of their potential impact on healthcare outcomes. This qualitative study seeks not to establish correlations but to explore underlying factors and nuances. This research investigates how the E-Health system can enhance nurses' job satisfaction and contribute to aftercare follow-up in Adult Medical Daycare in New Jersey, ultimately improving patient care. This research delves into the missed opportunities for aftercare follow-up in Adult Medical Daycare, New Jersey, aiming to enhance patient care effectiveness. Addressing the specific problem of the daycare's challenge in implementing aftercare follow-up, which leads to missed opportunities for more effective patient care, this study builds upon previous research that underscores the significance of consistent information provision to enhance user trust and utilization.

LITERATURE SUPPORT

ADVANCING THEORY

PROJECT TYPE & ORGANIZATION PERMISSION

PROJECT TYPE

This qualitative single case study will focus on investigating the role and impact of the E-Health system at an Adult Medical Daycare in the State of New Jersey. The study will examine the system's effectiveness in addressing the specific problem of patient aftercare follow-up, aiming to uncover potential benefits such as error reduction, enhanced patient safety, and improved communication. By exploring the implementation of the E-Health system in this context, the project aims to provide insights for enhancing patient care outcomes and addressing missed opportunities for effective aftercare follow-up. According to Mickan et al. (2019), the E-Health system is essential for communication in most healthcare facilities since, according to previous research, it can help reduce the risk of errors and improve patient safety by enhancing quick communication and medical response. The system enhances communication between patients and healthcare providers (Mickan et al.,

2019). Research on factors affecting Golden Years Care's daily operations can reveal critical elements contributing to challenges in integrating and adopting the E-Health system. The study can provide in-depth research since it offers a thorough analysis, produces better results, and applies knowledge to most other healthcare facilities (Mickan et al., 2019).

ORGANIZATION PERMISSION

RESEARCH QUESTIONS AND METHODOLOGY

RESEARCH QUESTION

1. What are the key factors contributing to the lack of aftercare follow-up for patients at Adult Medical Daycare in the State of New Jersey?
2. How can implementing an E-Health system enhance aftercare follow-up processes and improve overall patient care effectiveness at the Adult Medical Daycare in New Jersey?

METHODOLOGY

The selected research methodology for this study involved conducting a qualitative single case study, which proved highly appropriate for investigating the specific problem outlined in this research: the inability of the Adult Medical Daycare in the State of New Jersey to institute aftercare follow-up for patients, resulting in missed opportunities for delivering more effective patient care. The qualitative single case study approach allowed for an in-depth exploration of the complex and context-dependent challenges the Adult Medical Daycare faced in implementing aftercare follow-up practices.

The study aimed to uncover the unique organizational and contextual factors that contributed to the problem by focusing on a single case, the Golden Years Care facility. Gerring (2017) discussed that the qualitative nature of a methodology facilitates a nuanced understanding of the issue from the perspective of those directly involved. Interviews were conducted with the administrators of the Golden Years Care facility, enabling the collection of rich and detailed insights into the current aftercare follow-up practices, underlying barriers, and potential strategies for improvement. These interviews provided a window into the administrators' firsthand experiences and perspectives, shedding light on the intricate dynamics that influenced aftercare follow-up.

DATA COLLECTION

The chosen data collection method for this study, one-on-one semi-structured interviews, aligns well with the specific problem statement addressing the inability of the Adult Medical Daycare in the State of New Jersey to institute aftercare follow-up for patients. Using semi-structured interviews provides a comprehensive and in-depth exploration of staff members' experiences, opinions, and challenges related to the E-Health system and its potential impact on aftercare follow-up processes. Semi-structured interviews are particularly suitable for this study due to their flexibility in allowing participants to express themselves openly. As Bearman (2019) highlighted, this method encourages rich and contextual data collection, which is crucial for understanding the intricacies of aftercare follow-up practices and uncovering potential barriers to its effective implementation. Given the complexity of healthcare processes and the specific focus on aftercare follow-up, semi-structured interviews enable participants to elaborate on their unique perspectives, shedding light on nuances that quantitative data alone might miss.

The chosen data collection method also aligns with the qualitative nature of the study, which seeks to explore the underlying reasons for the identified problem. By engaging in in-depth conversations with staff members, researchers can delve into the intricate details of aftercare follow-up practices, identify any existing gaps or challenges, and gain insights into potential solutions. Roulston and Choi (2018) state that qualitative interviews offer the opportunity to capture participants' subjective experiences, allowing for a deeper understanding of their viewpoints and motivations. Furthermore, the semi-structured format of the interviews ensures a degree of consistency across interviews while also accommodating the exploration of diverse perspectives. This format enables the researcher to guide the discussion using open-ended questions related to the E-Health system and aftercare follow-up while allowing participants to introduce new insights or elaborate on specific points of interest. This balance between structure and flexibility enhances the credibility and rigor of the data collected (DeJonckheere & Vaughn, 2019).

DATA ANALYSIS

The selected approach for data analysis, which involves both narrative and thematic analysis, is particularly appropriate for addressing the specific problem of the inability of the Adult Medical Daycare in the State of New Jersey to institute aftercare follow-up for patients, ultimately leading to missed opportunities for delivering more effective patient care. Narrative analysis is a suitable method for delving into the participants' perspectives and experiences related to utilizing the E-Health system and the challenges they encounter in implementing aftercare follow-up. By allowing participants to share their narratives, this approach provides a comprehensive and detailed account of their viewpoints, shedding light on the intricacies of the problem. As Akinyode and Khan (2018) highlighted, narrative analysis facilitates a deep exploration of individual stories and helps researchers uncover rich insights into participants' experiences.

Thematic analysis is well-suited for identifying common patterns and themes that emerge from the collected data. This approach aligns intending to categorize significant themes related to the effectiveness and ineffectiveness of the E-Health system and its impact on aftercare follow-up. As described by Richards and Hemphill (2018), thematic analysis involves systematically organizing and analyzing data to identify recurring themes, providing a structured framework for understanding the complexities of the problem at hand. Considering the specific problem statement, narrative analysis will enable the researcher to capture the voices of healthcare professionals, administrators, and other relevant stakeholders involved in patient care and aftercare processes at the Adult Medical Daycare. Their narratives will offer valuable insights into their challenges in implementing aftercare follow-up and utilizing the E-Health system to its fullest potential.

Through narrative analysis, the researcher can gain a deeper understanding of the specific barriers and missed opportunities for effective patient care within the context of the Adult Medical Daycare. Subsequently, thematic analysis will allow the researcher to identify overarching themes that emerge from the narratives, potentially uncovering factors such as lack of training, resource constraints, communication gaps, or technological barriers contributing to the inability to effectively institute aftercare follow-up (Castleberry & Nolen, 2018). By categorizing and analyzing these themes, the study can provide a structured framework for addressing the problem and proposing targeted solutions to enhance the utilization of the E-Health system and improve patient care outcomes.

SECTION 2: LITERATURE SUPPORT

DESCRIPTION OF THE PROBLEM AND BUSINESS PRACTICES

DESCRIPTION OF THE PROBLEM

The problem addressed in this study revolves around the underutilization of E-Health systems in healthcare practices. E-Health systems, with their advanced technological capabilities, have the potential to revolutionize healthcare delivery and improve patient outcomes (Sneha & Straub, 2017). These systems enable healthcare professionals to access real-time patient data, track treatment progress, and collaborate seamlessly, leading to comprehensive and coordinated patient care. However, despite their significant advantages, there are indications that many healthcare practitioners are not fully embracing these systems, resulting in missed opportunities for timely interventions and communication gaps among providers.

In an optimized E-Health system, healthcare professionals can efficiently manage patient information, streamline administrative tasks, and enhance communication between departments. This leads to improved organizational efficiency and more time dedicated to direct patient care (Baumann et al., 2018). However, when staff members fail to utilize these systems, manual and inefficient processes adequately may persist, hindering the healthcare facility's ability to deliver optimal patient care and compromising overall organizational effectiveness. The underutilization of E-Health systems in healthcare practices calls for a focused investigation to understand the root causes and barriers faced by healthcare professionals. By gaining insights into the reasons for underutilization, healthcare facilities can develop targeted interventions to address these challenges effectively. Factors such as inadequate training, resistance to change, or concerns about data privacy and security may contribute to the reluctance of staff members to fully embrace the E-Health systems.

DESCRIPTION OF BUSINESS PRACTICES

E-Health systems encompass various digital tools and technologies designed to streamline healthcare operations, enhance patient care, and improve organizational efficiency. These practices can include adopting electronic health records (EHRs), telemedicine platforms, patient portals, wearable devices, and other digital tools to facilitate communication and data management. In healthcare settings, well-implemented E-Health systems can have transformative effects. For instance, EHRs enable healthcare professionals to access patients' medical records in real time, leading to more informed decision-making, enhanced care coordination, and improved patient safety.

Telemedicine platforms allow for remote patient consultations, expanding access to healthcare services, particularly in underserved areas. Patient portals offer a means for patients to interact with their healthcare providers, schedule appointments, access lab results, and gain access to educational resources (Kataria & Ravindran, 2020). Understanding the dynamics of E-Health system utilization in healthcare practices and identifying the factors leading to missed opportunities for aftercare follow-up in the Adult Medical Daycare setting is crucial for addressing the specific problem statement. By recognizing these challenges, organizations can develop targeted interventions and strategies to foster successful adoption, improve patient care, and enhance organizational effectiveness.

DISCUSSION ON PREVIOUS RESEARCH

The problem addressed in this study is the underutilization of E-Health services in healthcare practices, exacerbated by employee resistance to organizational change. This is particularly evident in the inability of the Adult Medical Daycare in the State of New Jersey to institute aftercare follow-up for patients. Both of these issues can have significant negative impacts on the respective industries. In the healthcare sector, implementing E-Health systems has become a strategic initiative to improve patient care and organizational efficiency (Al-Radaideh & Alazzam, 2020). Inefficient utilization of these systems can disrupt workflows and lead to increased administrative burden, hampering the organization's ability to provide optimal patient care.

Inefficient utilization of these systems can disrupt workflows and lead to increased administrative burden, hampering the organization's ability to provide optimal patient care. Previous research on E-Health system utilization in healthcare practices has identified various factors influencing healthcare professionals' adoption of these systems. Inadequate training and technical support, data privacy and security concerns, and resistance to change are among the key issues hindering effective utilization. Studies have shown that healthcare practitioners who receive proper training and support are more likely to embrace E-Health systems and leverage their capabilities for improved patient care (Maksimović & Vujović, 2017).

To address the underutilization of E-Health services in healthcare practices, providing comprehensive training and technical support to healthcare professionals is essential. Engaging staff members in the decision-making process during system implementation can foster a sense of ownership and increase buy-in. Addressing data privacy and security concerns through robust information governance measures can build trust and encourage data sharing among healthcare professionals. This study aims to bridge the gap between previous research findings and practical applications by providing tailored recommendations to address the identified problems. By understanding the unique context of healthcare businesses, this study seeks to contribute to improved patient care outcomes and organizational effectiveness in the retail clothing industry.

RESEARCH FRAMEWORK

The conceptual framework for this qualitative study is based on the Technology Acceptance Model (TAM) theory developed by Fred Davis (1989). The TAM theory aims to provide insights into how users accept and adopt new technologies. In this research, we will utilize the framework to investigate the factors that influence the acceptance and utilization of the E-Health system within Golden Years Care facility.

KEY TENETS OF THE TECHNOLOGY ACCEPTANCE MODEL (TAM)

- **Perceived Usefulness:** According to TAM, users are more likely to accept and use technology if they perceive it as useful in enhancing their performance or making tasks easier (Taherdoost, 2018).
- **Perceived Ease of Use:** According to Taherdoost (2018), TAM also emphasizes the importance of perceived ease of use, where users are more inclined to adopt a technology if they perceive it as easy to learn and use.

CONNECTION TO THE STUDY APPROACH AND RESEARCH QUESTIONS

TAM provides a framework for understanding how healthcare facility staff accept and integrate the E-Health system (Taher-doost, 2018). By examining staff perceptions of the E-Health system's usefulness in improving their tasks and its ease of use, this study can assess the factors that influence staff members' decision to adopt or resist the technology. Understanding staff attitudes towards these factors is crucial for identifying barriers to adoption and designing effective strategies for implementation.

RELEVANCE TO INSTRUMENT DEVELOPMENT AND DATA ANALYSIS

The conceptual framework informs the development of interview questions and data analysis. The interview questions will be designed to explore staff members' perceptions of the perceived usefulness and ease of use of the E-Health system. The responses will then be analyzed to identify patterns and themes related to staff members' attitudes and beliefs about the E-Health system's potential benefits and usability. This approach aligns with TAM's focus on users' perceptions and attitudes as key determinants of technology adoption (Taher-doost, 2018). By applying the TAM theory, this study aims to uncover insights that can guide the successful implementation of the E-Health system at Golden Years Care facility.

Figure 1: Framework Diagram

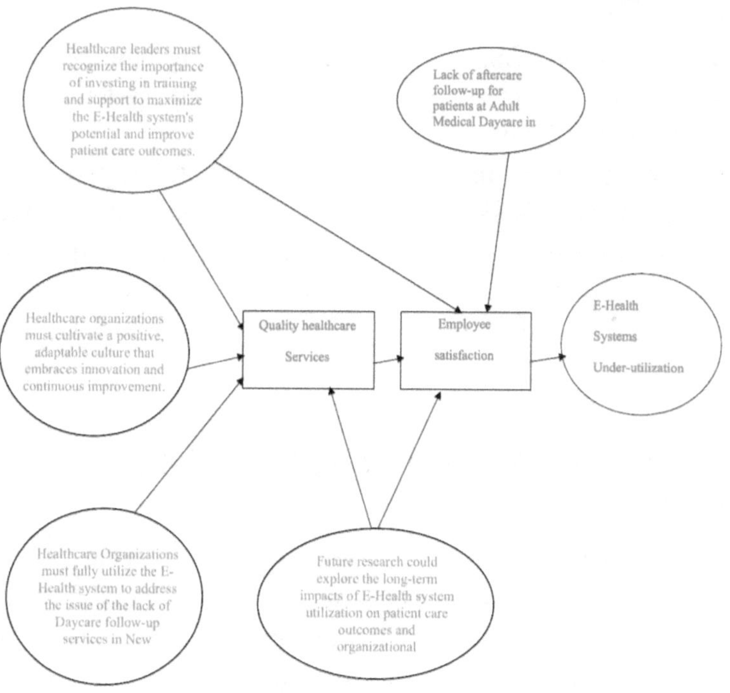

Introduction

The framework diagram is a visual tool to elucidate our research study's intricate relationships among core elements. It visually depicts how concepts, theories, actors, and constructs interact to shape the investigation's scope and outcomes (Collins & Stockton, 2018). The purpose of this diagram is to provide a comprehensive understanding of the dynamics at play within our study.

Diagram

The diagram showcases the dynamic interactions and flow

of information and action among the central components of the research framework. By providing a visual overview of the relationships between concepts, theories, actors, and constructs, the diagram enhances our grasp of the interconnected nature of these elements.

Concepts

Perceived Ease of Use: Based on TAM, this concept explores how healthcare professionals perceive the ease of using E-Health systems.

Perceived Usefulness: Another key TAM element is that this concept delves into how healthcare professionals perceive the effectiveness and benefits of E-Health systems.

Theories

Technology Acceptance Model (TAM): TAM, a cornerstone of the study, outlines the factors influencing individuals' acceptance and utilization of new technologies. Perceived ease of use and usefulness are key elements within TAM guiding the exploration (Taherdoost, 2018).

Actors

Healthcare Professionals: The primary actors in the present study, healthcare professionals, including doctors and nurses, play a central role in adopting and using E-Health systems.

Constructs

Behavioral Intention to Use: Rooted in TAM, this construct reflects how healthcare professionals express their intention to use E-Health systems.

Actual Use Behavior: This construct captures the actual

utilization of E-Health systems by healthcare professionals in their daily practices.

Relationship Between Concepts, Theories, Actors, and Constructs

The framework illustrates the alignment between concepts and constructs within the TAM. Perceived ease of use and perceived usefulness influence healthcare professionals' behavioral intention to use E-Health systems (Wahyuni, 2017). This intention, in turn, shapes the actual use behavior, reflecting the impact of TAM on the practices of healthcare professionals.

Summary

The framework diagram presents a holistic view of how concepts, theories, actors, and constructs interact. Focused on the TAM theory, the diagram highlights the relationships between perceived ease of use, perceived usefulness, behavioral intention to use, and actual use behavior within the context of healthcare professionals and E-Health systems.

This comprehensive visual representation guides the exploration of the factors influencing the adoption and utilization of E-Health systems.

Summary of Literature Support

The conceptual framework for this qualitative study was based on the Technology Acceptance Model (TAM) theory proposed by Davis in 1989. This theory provided a structured foundation for comprehending how individuals perceive and integrate new technologies, like E-Health systems, into their work environments. By employing this framework, the investigation aimed to uncover the factors influencing the adoption and utilization of the E-Health system within healthcare practices.

The fundamental tenets of the Technology Acceptance Model, encompassing perceived ease of use and perceived usefulness, closely aligned with the study's approach and research inquiries. The examination of healthcare staff's perceptions regarding the system's ease of use and its utility in their daily responsibilities yielded valuable insights into impediments to adoption and avenues for enhancement. Moreover, the TAM theory underlined that attitudes toward technology adoption directly shaped behavioral intentions and actual usage (Wahyuni, 2017). This facet facilitated the exploration of how healthcare staff's attitudes toward the E-Health system influenced their readiness to embrace the technology. Consequently, this insight informed the development of customized strategies to address varying attitudes and levels of acceptance.

COMPLETE LITERATURE REVIEW

INTRODUCTION

In this chapter, we present a comprehensive literature review that builds upon the problem and purpose of the study outlined in Chapter 1. The study examines the effectiveness of the E-Health system, focusing on healthcare professionals' utilization factors that are aligned with the specific problem of patient aftercare gaps in New Jersey's Adult Medical Daycare. The literature review concisely summarizes current research on E-Health systems, technology adoption in healthcare settings, and factors influencing system effectiveness. By examining the existing literature, we establish the problem's relevance and identify gaps that this study intends to address. Through this comprehensive literature review, we aim to develop the significance of our research in contributing to theory advancement and practice improvements, as well as filling the gap in the current literature related to E-Health system effectiveness in healthcare settings.

LITERATURE SEARCH STRATEGY

To conduct a comprehensive literature review, this research project utilized various library databases and search engines to access current and seminal literature on the E-Health system's effectiveness in healthcare settings. The primary focus was to gather sources published within the last five years to ensure the relevance and currency of the information

obtained. The following are the accessed library databases and search engines, along with the key search terms used for the literature search:

PubMed: This database was utilized to search for articles from reputable medical journals. Key search terms included: "E-Health system," "healthcare technology," "healthcare informatics," "EHR adoption," "E-Health benefits," "E-Health challenges," and "E-Health patient outcomes." **ScienceDirect:** ScienceDirect was used to access various scientific research articles. Key search terms included: "E-Health implementation," "healthcare professionals and E-Health," "E-Health communication," "E-Health and patient safety," "E-Health usability," and "E-Health user satisfaction."

Google Scholar: Google Scholar was used to supplement the search with additional sources, including conference papers, theses, and other scholarly materials. Key search terms included: "E-Health system effectiveness," "E-Health adoption," "E-Health utilization," "E-Health barriers," and "E-Health success factors."

IEEE Xplore: This database was consulted to access relevant research articles related to technology in healthcare settings. Key search terms included: "E-Health technology," "healthcare IT systems," "E-Health innovations," "E-Health security," and "E-Health data privacy."

Embase: Embase was included to search for articles from biomedical literature and conference proceedings. Key search terms had: "E-Health outcomes," "E-Health implementation challenges," "E-Health impact on patient care," "E-Health user experience," and "E-Health data analytics."

The search strategy incorporated various combinations of the key search terms using the Boolean operators "AND" and "OR" to broaden or narrow the search scope as needed.

Truncation and wildcards were also used to account for different variations of the terms. An example search strategy could be: ("E-Health system" OR "healthcare technology") AND ("implementation" OR "adoption" OR "utilization") AND ("patient outcomes" OR "user satisfaction" OR "communication").

To ensure that all relevant literature was included, the search strategy was not limited to specific geographical regions but instead focused on the broader context of E-Health system implementation and utilization in healthcare settings. Additionally, the search was limited to English-language publications to ensure better comprehension and analysis of the gathered data. The initial literature search produced many articles, conference papers, and other sources. The selection process included assessing each source's relevance, credibility, and quality. Only peer-reviewed articles and scholarly materials that met the study's objectives were retained for further analysis. Key seminal literature related to the adoption and impact of E-Health systems in healthcare settings was also included to provide a foundation for understanding the research topic's historical development and key findings.

In cases where there was limited current research, or few recent dissertations and conference proceedings available, efforts were made to contact experts in the field, consult relevant professional organizations, or access government reports and white papers related to E-Health system implementation and outcomes. This approach allowed the research project to ensure a comprehensive and up-to-date literature review, even in areas where current research was scarce. The literature search strategy adopted for this research project ensured the collection of relevant, high-quality sources to provide a comprehensive overview of the current state of knowledge regarding the effectiveness and challenges of E-Health systems in healthcare settings.

THEORETICAL FOUNDATION

THEORY: THE TECHNOLOGY ACCEPTANCE MODEL (TAM)

THEORETICAL BACKGROUND

TAM is a widely used theory in information systems and technology adoption. It was initially proposed by Fred Davis in 1989. The TAM is grounded in social psychology and behavioral theories and seeks to explain how users' attitudes and beliefs influence their acceptance and adoption of new technologies.

KEY CONCEPTS AND PROPOSITIONS

TAM is based on two key beliefs: perceived usefulness (PU) and perceived ease of use (PEOU). According to TAM, users' intentions to use technology depend on their perceptions of its usefulness and ease of use (Wahyuni, 2017).

Perceived Usefulness (PU): PU refers to the user's belief that a particular technology will enhance their performance and productivity in achieving specific goals. As stated by Wahyuni (2017), users are more likely to adopt a technology if they perceive it as helpful in accomplishing their tasks.

Perceived Ease of Use (PEOU): PEOU refers to the user's

belief that a technology is easy to use and requires minimal effort to understand and operate. Users are more likely to adopt technologies perceived as easy to use (Wahyuni, 2017).

The TAM proposes that PU and PEOU directly influence users' attitudes toward using the technology, which, in turn, affects their intention to use the technology. Ultimately, these attitudes and intentions shape the actual use behavior of the technology.

LITERATURE ANALYSIS

The Technology Acceptance Model has been widely applied in various fields, including healthcare, to understand the adoption and acceptance of new technologies. Here are four relevant studies that have utilized TAM:

Study 1: A study by Nguyen et al. (2020) applied TAM to investigate the acceptance of telemedicine among healthcare professionals. The study found that perceived usefulness and ease of use significantly influenced healthcare professionals' intention to adopt telemedicine for remote consultations.

Study 2: In a study by Tubaishat (2017), TAM was employed to examine the adoption of electronic health records (EHR) in a hospital setting. The research revealed that perceived ease of use and usefulness significantly influenced the nurses' intention to adopt EHR for patient documentation.

Study 3: A study by Alhassan et al. (2017) used TAM to explore the adoption of Mobil E-Health applications among patients with chronic diseases. The findings demonstrated that patients' perception of the apps' usefulness and ease of use significantly influenced their intention to adopt and use them for managing their health.

Study 4: In a study by Kivekäs et al. (2018), TAM was utilized to examine the acceptance of a computerized physician order entry system in a healthcare organization. The study revealed that the system's perceived usefulness and ease of use significantly impacted physicians' intention to prescribe it for medication.

THE RATIONALE FOR THEORY CHOICE

The TAM Model is particularly relevant to the present study as it focuses on users' perceptions and attitudes toward adopting a new technology, which aligns with the study's objective of understanding the effectiveness and adoption challenges of the E-Health system. By applying TAM, the researcher can gain insights into the healthcare professionals' beliefs regarding the system's usefulness in enhancing patient care and ease of use in their daily workflow. TAM's emphasis on users' attitudes and intentions can inform the study's design by guiding the formulation of interview questions and data analysis (Wahyuni, 2017).

Understanding how healthcare professionals perceive the E-Health system's usefulness and ease of use can help identify barriers and facilitators to its adoption and implementation within the healthcare facility.

RELATIONSHIP WITH THE PRESENT STUDY

The present study aims to explore the adoption and impact of the E-Health system at a healthcare facility. TAM directly relates to this study as it provides a framework to analyze the factors influencing healthcare professionals' intention to adopt and use the E-Health system. The research questions of this study relate to TAM's major propositions as they focus on understanding healthcare professionals' perceptions of the system's usefulness in enhancing patient care and their perceptions of its ease of use in their daily tasks (Wahyuni, 2017) By exploring these perceptions, the study aims to determine the factors that influence the system's adoption within the facility, building upon the existing theory of TAM.

Moreover, the study challenges TAM's assumptions to some

extent by examining the specific context of the healthcare facility and the unique challenges and opportunities associated with adopting the E-Health system. The research explores how social influences, training, and

support within the facility may shape healthcare professionals' attitudes toward the system's adoption. TAM provides a robust theoretical foundation for the present study, offering a comprehensive framework to understand healthcare professionals' perceptions and attitudes toward the E-Health system's adoption (Wahyuni, 2017). By applying the model, the study can identify critical factors influencing adoption, guide data collection and analysis, and inform strategies for enhancing the system's effectiveness and acceptance within the healthcare facility.

LITERATURE REVIEW

The introduction of E-Health systems in hospital settings can change how outpatient tracking and communication are handled, leading to improved patient care and overall hospital efficiency. In this literature review, the researcher will examine the role of E-Health systems in enhancing the tracking and communication of outpatients within hospital environments. By studying research papers in this field, the goal is to determine the strengths and weaknesses of different approaches and justify why certain variables and concepts are chosen for implementation. Through an analysis of existing literature, the study aims to provide insights into the current knowledge, controversies, and gaps within this research area.

One of the benefits of E-Health systems is their ability to offer real-time updates on patient's conditions. According to Bauer (2018), this feature allows healthcare providers to closely monitor patients' progress, enabling them to intervene in case of any changes or concerning patterns. This continuous exchange of information between patients and healthcare providers enhances the coordination of care. Enables healthcare teams to make well-informed decisions without delay. By addressing patients' needs and concerns, hospitals can effectively prevent potential complications, decrease hospital readmission rates, and improve overall patient care outcomes.

The enhanced communication facilitated by E-Health systems plays a role in establishing trust and promoting patient engagement. As highlighted by Raj et al. (2017), involved patients who maintain open lines of communication with their healthcare providers are more likely to follow treatment plans diligently and actively participate in managing their health. E-Health systems grant patients access to their health information, personalized treatment plans, and educational resources, empowering them to take control of their health journey and make informed decisions about their care.

The utilization of E-Health systems impacts the efficiency of hospital services.

These systems enable communication and information sharing, resulting in a reduced administrative workload for healthcare professionals. This, in turn, allows them to focus on providing care to patients. By automating tasks like scheduling appointments, delivering test results, and sending medication reminders, E-Health systems effectively save time for healthcare professionals. Consequently, they can dedicate attention to individual patients and complex medical cases. Integrating E-Health systems with health records (EHRs) ensures seamless data exchanges and access to comprehensive patient information. This integration guarantees that healthcare providers have an understanding of patients' medical backgrounds. As a result, accurate diagnoses can be made, enabling tailored treatment plans to be developed. Ultimately, this personalized approach contributes to improved health outcomes and higher levels of patient satisfaction.

Despite the advantages offered by E-Health systems, it is essential to acknowledge the challenges associated with their successful implementation. Bauer (2018) highlights data privacy and security issues and the initial investment required for adopting and integrating these technologies into existing hospital systems. Healthcare organizations must proactively address

these challenges by implementing data protection measures and ensuring compliance with healthcare regulations and standards. E-Health systems have brought about a transformation in the field of healthcare by centralizing patient information and facilitating seamless communication between healthcare providers and patients. The adoption of E-Health systems has proven to be highly advantageous in improving patient care and optimizing hospital operations. These systems offer healthcare professionals access to vital patient data, enabling faster decision making, ultimately leading to better treatment outcomes and higher patient satisfaction.

In a study conducted by Alazzam et al. (2021), the impact of E-Health systems on outpatient treatment progress and overall hospital efficiency was further explored. The findings revealed a relationship between the implementation of E-Health systems and enhanced hospital efficiency. With the presence of these systems, healthcare providers can monitor the progress of patients' treatment in time, ensuring timely interventions and adjustments to treatment plans whenever necessary. This proactive approach contributes to improved patient outcomes and streamlines workflows within the hospital, optimizing resource utilization and minimizing unnecessary delays.

In addition to improving hospital operations, E-Health systems play a role in tracking patients, especially those receiving outpatient care. According to Anshari et al. (2021), leveraging E-Health systems is crucial for enhancing hospital monitoring. By integrating these systems into healthcare services, medical professionals can track patients' progress effectively, ensuring they diligently follow their treatment plans. Continuous monitoring allows healthcare providers to identify any deviations from the course of treatment and promptly address potential issues, ultimately leading to improved patient outcomes and overall healthcare quality.

Effective communication through E-Health platforms emerges as a component in tracking and supporting outpatients while ensuring their treatment progress stays on track. According to Andersen et al. (2018), establishing communication between patients and healthcare providers is essential for building trust and promoting patient engagement in their own care. E-Health communication tools like messaging platforms and telemedicine facilitate regular interactions between patients and healthcare professionals, enabling patients to provide updates on their health status and seek clarifications about their treatment plans. Consequently, healthcare providers can offer personalized guidance and support, resulting in adherence to treatments and better health outcomes.

Moreover, E-Health communication plays a role in educating and empowering patients. The availability of resources and information through E-Health platforms allows individuals to actively participate in managing their health. This increased engagement improves self-care and decision-making and contributes to the overall progress of treatments and well-being. Effective communication strategies in outpatient care within hospital services are crucial, as Tremoulet et al. (2020) emphasized. Tailored approaches like telemedicine and secure messaging platforms enable hospitals to maintain contact with outpatients, ensuring continuity of care and enhancing patient satisfaction. By addressing concerns, monitoring treatment progress, and providing timely support, healthcare providers cultivate more robust relationships with their patients. Ultimately, this leads to social change by improving accessibility to healthcare services and enhancing patient outcomes.

Integrating E-Health systems in healthcare settings has implications for positive social change. Sharikh et al. (2020) discussed utilizing E-Health systems for hospital client tracking has improved outcomes and overall healthcare quality. Implementing tracking mechanisms

hospitals can ensure that patients who are not admitted

receive prompt medical interventions. This proactive approach reduces the chances of complications and readmissions. Moreover, E-Health systems enable healthcare providers to monitor patients and intervene swiftly whenever necessary. This enhances the quality of patient care and improves the overall efficiency and effectiveness of healthcare services.

The use of E-Health systems has the potential to overcome barriers and enhance access to healthcare, especially in remote or underserved areas, as highlighted by Miah et al. (2017) in their comprehensive analysis. These systems allow patients to access healthcare services from the comfort of their homes, thereby reducing unnecessary hospital visits and minimizing travel expenses. This aspect becomes more significant in regions where healthcare infrastructure is limited as E-Health systems can assist in extending medical services to individuals who may otherwise face challenges in obtaining adequate healthcare.

The cost-effectiveness of implementing E-Health systems within hospital settings is another factor that contributes to positive social change. According to Massoudi et al. (2019), hospitals can efficiently manage outpatient care by leveraging monitoring and telemedicine capabilities to reduce the frequency of hospital visits for routine checkups. This optimization of resources leads to decreased healthcare costs and better allocation of healthcare resources, ultimately benefiting healthcare providers and patients. Moreover, the cost-effectiveness offered by E-Health systems enables healthcare organizations to reallocate their resources toward enhancing patient care and investing in medical technologies.

E-Health communication also has a significant impact on enhancing the effectiveness of hospital services through improved outpatient tracking. Zhang et al. (2019) discussed how better outpatient tracking can result in fewer treatment delays and

complications, leading to cost savings for both hospitals and patients. By using E-Health systems for tracking, healthcare providers can closely monitor patients' progress, identify any deviations from the treatment plan, and intervene promptly when necessary. This proactive approach to outpatient tracking improves patient outcomes and reduces the need for costly and avoidable interventions, ultimately leading to cost savings for healthcare facilities and patients alike.

E-Health systems have emerged as a powerful tool to improve patient safety and reduce medical errors. Susanto and Chen (2017) delve into utilizing E-Health systems for patient tracking and highlight the benefits and challenges of implementing such systems effectively. One of the key advantages of E-Health systems is their ability to provide real-time alerts and reminders to healthcare providers. These alerts can range from medication adherence prompts to allergy alerts and potential drug interactions. By receiving timely alerts, healthcare providers can avoid possible medical errors and adverse events, ensuring patient safety and delivering high-quality care.

Real-time access to data through E-Health systems is crucial for healthcare professionals to make informed decisions and ensure safer care delivery. According to a study conducted by Susanto and Chen (2017), having comprehensive and up-to-date patient information empowers healthcare providers to make accurate treatment plans, administer medications effectively, and coordinate care efficiently. This not only enhances patient safety but also improves healthcare delivery's overall efficiency and effectiveness. These safety measures act as layers of protection, significantly reducing the risks associated with medication errors and adverse drug reactions. By prioritizing safety when designing E-Health systems, healthcare facilities can

ensure that patient tracking and communication processes enhance healthcare quality and improve patient outcomes.

E-Health systems play a role in promoting patient empowerment and involvement in healthcare decision-making. By granting patients access to their health records, treatment progress updates, and personalized care plans, these systems empower individuals to manage their well-being. According to a study conducted by Dymyt and Dymyt (2018), when patients have real-time access to health information through E-Health systems, they tend to become more engaged in their treatment plans and adhere better to prescribed therapies. This sense of empowerment results in health outcomes as patients become more knowledgeable and engaged participants in their own care. Additionally, E-Health communication strategies have proven effective for outpatient monitoring within hospital services. Ammenwerth et al. (2019) stress that interactive communication platforms like patient portals facilitate seamless communication between patients and healthcare providers. Such channels of communication foster a sense of empowerment among patients, making them feel more involved in the decision-making process regarding their care. Patients can openly discuss concerns, ask questions and provide feedback all contributing to shared decision making and patient-centered care.

In alignment with a data-driven approach, Dash et al. (2019) delved into how E-Health communication influences the quality of hospital services and outpatient tracking. E-Health systems capture information about patient interactions, treatment progress, and outcomes. This wealth of data can be leveraged to evaluate performance and drive quality improvement efforts. By analyzing this information, healthcare organizations can identify areas that require enhancement while implementing evidence-based practices to enhance overall patient experiences. As a result, the healthcare environment becomes streamlined, patient-centric centric, and dedicated to delivering high-quality care.

The incorporation of E-Health systems in healthcare services has the potential to bring about a transformation in patient care. It empowers patients to improve communication and enables data-driven decision-making. However, there are still challenges that need to be addressed. One primary concern is ensuring the privacy and security of data. As E-Health systems gather and store information, it is crucial to implement strong data protection measures and adhere to privacy regulations to safeguard patient data. Additionally, successful implementation requires healthcare organizations to invest in training and support for both healthcare professionals and patients. Highlighting the involvement and collaboration of staff during the implementation process can foster acceptance and enthusiasm for using E-Health systems in practice.

E-Health systems are further essential in enhancing communication and collaboration among healthcare providers, leading to better patient outcomes and reduced treatment delays. A study by Tebeje and Klein (2021) explored the impact of E-communication on monitoring outpatient progress in hospitals, especially during the COVID–19 Pandemic. The findings emphasized that E-Health systems facilitate communication among healthcare teams involved in a patient's care. With access to real-time patient data and practical communication tools, healthcare providers can exchange information quickly and securely. Honest time communication guarantees that every team member is well-informed, allowing them to work together efficiently. Consequently, patients benefit from a well-coordinated healthcare experience, ultimately improving their treatment results.

In addition to improving communication, E-Health systems also simplify the exchange of information among healthcare providers, ultimately making hospital services more efficient.

Haleem et al. (2021) conducted a study to examine how E-Health systems impact outpatient treatment progress and hospitals' efficiency. The research revealed that E-Health systems offer a platform where healthcare providers can access patient information, test results, and treatment plans. This easy accessibility leads to decision-making and reduced treatment delays, ultimately enhancing the overall efficiency of hospital services. Healthcare teams can collaborate effectively by facilitating communication channels, resulting in improved patient care and satisfaction.

Continuity of care is another aspect that E-Health systems promote. According to Kim and Lee (2021), E-Health systems are utilized to enhance client tracking in hospitals. The study emphasizes that these systems enable the sharing of patient data across different healthcare facilities. This ensures that all healthcare providers have access to information regardless of where they seek medical attention. Consequently, patients receive uninterrupted care as all healthcare professionals are well-informed about their medical history and ongoing treatments. This consistent and uninterrupted provision of healthcare not only enhances the well-being of patients but also lowers the chances of medical mistakes and unnecessary tests, resulting in more effective and economical healthcare services.

Communication in the field of E-Health plays a role in tracking and supporting outpatient services. According to Alexandru and Ianculescu (2019), there is potential in using E-Health systems to create personalized care plans and patient-centered approaches. These systems can be tailored to meet individual patients' needs, preferences, and requirements. By doing so, healthcare providers can ensure that the care they provide aligns with each patient's unique characteristics, goals, and values. This approach fosters levels of patient satisfaction and engagement, as individuals feel more involved in the decision-making process and empowered to manage their own health actively. In addition, E-Health systems have emerged as tools for improving patient safety and reducing medical errors within hospital services.

Research conducted by Barbosa and Dal Sasso (2022), and Mshali et al. (2018) sheds light on how accurate time monitoring and error detection capabilities inherent in E-tracking can contribute to enhanced patient safety. In the study conducted by Barbosa and Dal Sasso (2022), the researchers focused on how E-Health tracking can improve hospital services for outpatients.

One of their findings highlighted the valuable role of E-Health systems in providing real-time alerts for potential medical errors or adverse events. By monitoring patient data, these systems can automatically detect any abnormalities or deviations from the expected parameters. Prompt notifications are then sent to healthcare providers, enabling them to intervene and address issues before they escalate and cause harm to patients. For example, E-Health systems can flag vital signs, discrepancies in medication records, or missed follow-up appointments. This immediate alerting mechanism significantly enhances safety by allowing proactive measures to mitigate potential risks.

Likewise, Mshali et al. (2018) conducted a review of various studies that aimed to assess the impact of E-Health tracking on outpatient care. The review demonstrated that when equipped with error detection algorithms, E-Health systems can play a role in reducing medical errors. Automating the process of error detection and flagging these systems help. Rectify errors related to medication administration, treatment protocols, and documentation. For instance, E-Health systems can compare medications with a patient's known allergies and current medications, preventing potential harmful interactions. Additionally, these systems can confirm that healthcare providers adhere to evidence-based treatment guidelines, guaranteeing that patients receive secure care. By simplifying the identification and resolution of errors, E-Health systems help in creating a safer healthcare setting and ultimately improve patient outcomes.

In addition to enhancing safety, E-Health systems also play a crucial role in supporting data-driven decision-making and quality improvement efforts within hospital settings. The studies conducted by Iqbal et al. (2019) and Ratwani (2017) highlight the potential of E-Health systems in generating valuable data and insights that can inform healthcare practices. The study Iqbal et al. (2019) carried out focused on using E-Health systems for tracking patients and the associated benefits and challenges involved. These systems collect a range of data encompassing various aspects of patient care, hospital operations, and resource usage. This information includes demographics, treatment history, medication administration records, and laboratory results, among others. Healthcare facilities can effectively utilize this data to make informed patient care and resource allocation decisions. For instance, E-Health systems can provide real-time updates on bed availability, which helps hospitals optimize bed allocation while efficiently managing the flow of patients. Furthermore, these systems enable tracking outcomes and satisfaction scores—empowering healthcare administrators to identify areas that require improvement and implement initiatives to enhance overall quality.

Similarly, in the study by Ratwani (2017), which analyzed various E-Health communication strategies for outpatient tracking, E-Health systems were recognized for their data analytics and reporting capabilities. These systems can capture and analyze vast amounts of patient data, allowing hospitals to monitor key performance indicators (KPIs) related to patient care, efficiency, and safety. By tracking KPIs, hospitals can identify trends and patterns, measure the impact of interventions, and compare performance against benchmarks or industry standards. This data-driven approach empowers healthcare administrators to make evidence-based decisions and implement best practices to optimize patient care and hospital operations.

Patient engagement is crucial in healthcare, as actively involved patients are more likely to adhere to treatment plans and experience better health outcomes. E-Health technology is vital in enhancing patient engagement by providing patients with access to their health information, treatment plans, and personalized health data. Coughlin et al. (2017) emphasize that when patients have easy access to their medical records and health data through E-Health systems, they become more empowered to take charge of their health. This empowerment leads to better self-management and treatment adherence, improving patient outcomes.

Similarly, Anshari et al. (2021) delve into the impact of E-Health tracking on empowerment within hospital services. The availability of real-time health data through E-Health systems empowers patients to participate actively in their care decisions and make informed choices. By monitoring their health progress, tracking signs, and receiving personalized feedback, patients develop a sense of responsibility for their own well-being. Consequently, they are more likely to adopt behaviors and adhere to prescribed treatment plans, resulting in improved treatment outcomes and decreased healthcare expenditures.

Besides enhancing patient engagement, E-Health systems potentially transform communication between healthcare providers and patients. In the study by Santana et al. (2018), the focus lies on utilizing E-Health systems for monitoring outpatient progress and facilitating communication. The authors highlight how time data collection and communication encourage seamless interaction between healthcare professionals and patients. Through messaging platforms, telemedicine consultations, and patient portals enable continuous communication that allows healthcare providers to monitor patients' progress while promptly intervening remotely when necessary. This dynamic means of communication leads to developing treatment plans that ultimately result in enhanced patient care.

The impact of health (E-Health) systems on the workflow and quality of patient care has been extensively discussed in the literature. Kelly et al. (2020) examine how the implementation of E-Health systems affects hospital processes. These systems streamline data collection and communication, improving efficiency in workflow by reducing tasks and allowing healthcare professionals to dedicate more time to direct patient care. Furthermore, Dymyt (2020) discusses that E-Health systems contribute to coordination of care, decreased occurrences of medical errors, and enhanced patient safety. By consolidating information into a single accessible platform these systems empower healthcare professionals to make well-informed decisions, ultimately resulting in positive patient outcomes.

In addition to their impact on efficiency, E-Health communication plays a vital role in promoting patient-centered care. Alpert et al. (2017) delve into how communication through E-Health systems fosters strong relationships between patients and healthcare providers while also facilitating patient-centered decision-making processes. When patients can easily communicate with their healthcare professionals and actively participate in their treatment plans, they feel more involved in their care journey. This approach centered around patients leads to levels of satisfaction among patients and improved overall healthcare outcomes.

Expanding on the significance of E-Health communication tools within hospital services, Laukka et al. (2020) discusses tools employed for outpatient tracking purposes. There are tools available for communication in the healthcare industry, such as secure messaging platforms, telemedicine consultations and patient portals. Each of these tools has its own advantages and challenges, and hospitals should customize their communication strategies to fit patient preferences and technological capabilities. By identifying the suitable communication tools for different patient groups, hospitals can improve patient satisfaction and enhance the overall healthcare experience.

Despite the advantages of E-Health technology, particular challenges must be tackled to ensure its successful implementation. The literature has highlighted concerns regarding data privacy and security as E-Health systems involve the gathering and storing of patient information. Coventry and Branley (2018) delve into the considerations surrounding the use of E-Health systems for patient tracking. They recommend that it is imperative to safeguard data and ensure confidentiality to foster trust among patients and meet regulatory requirements.

Therefore, it is crucial to implement measures for data

protection that address these concerns while ensuring E-Health systems' safe and secure utilization.

To further enhance patient outcomes, researchers have explored how artificial intelligence (AI) and predictive analytics can be integrated into E-Health systems. Thomas., et al. (2021) discuss the potential of AI in analyzing data and predicting treatment responses. AI-driven E-Health systems can assist healthcare professionals in making precise diagnoses and treatment decisions, ultimately leading to improved patient outcomes. By utilizing AI algorithms, these E-Health systems can also identify high-risk patients. Intervene proactively to prevent adverse events. This innovative approach driven by AI holds promise for revolutionizing healthcare in the future.

Wearable devices have also attracted attention in the research as a tool for E-Health systems. In a study by Abuwarda et al. (2022), they explore how wearable devices can be integrated into E-Health systems to monitor patients in real-time. These devices can track signs, physical activity, and other health metrics, providing continuous data that healthcare professionals can use to monitor patient progress and make necessary adjustments to treatment plans. By incorporating devices into E-Health systems, remote patient monitoring becomes possible, especially for individuals in remote or rural areas, ultimately improving access to healthcare services.

Furthermore, telemedicine has been recognized as a component of E-Health systems for remotely tracking patients. In a study conducted by Haleem et al. (2021), they investigated the combined use of telemedicine and E-Health systems to enable patient monitoring and consultations. Telemedicine allows healthcare providers to assess patients virtually, discuss treatment plans, and offer support regardless of distance. This is particularly beneficial for individuals residing in remote regions as it enhances their access to specialized care and reduces the need for frequent in-person visits.

By reviewing and synthesizing studies related to key variables in the literature, we have gained valuable insights into how E-Health technology impacts patient engagement, treatment progress, hospital workflow, and patient centered care. Based on the data, the E-Health systems are essential in encouraging patient engagement. These systems empower individuals by granting them access to their health information and providing feedback. When patients actively utilize E-Health systems, they tend to adhere to treatment plans, ultimately resulting in improved health outcomes.

Electronic health (E-Health) systems play a role in facilitating seamless communication between healthcare providers and patients. They enable accurate time exchange of data and the creation of treatment plans. Integrating intelligence (AI) and predictive analytics in E-Health systems further enhance patient outcomes by assisting healthcare professionals in making well-informed decisions and identifying high-risk patients for timely interventions. In addition, devices and telemedicine complement E-Health systems by offering remote patient monitoring options and improving access to healthcare services, especially in remote or underserved areas.

While the existing literature demonstrates the benefits of E-Health technology, it also emphasizes the need to address particular challenges. Protecting patient data privacy and security requires robust measures to safeguard sensitive information. Ethical considerations, data protection, and obtaining consent should always be at the forefront of E-Health implementations. Despite the advancements made in E-Health technology, there are still gaps in the literature that require research. For instance, understanding the long-term impact of E-Health systems on engagement and treatment progress necessitates thorough exploration. Longitudinal studies tracking outcomes and adherence over extended periods will shed light on the sustainability and effectiveness of E-Health interventions. Additionally, conducting research focusing on patient populations across various healthcare settings will ensure that findings are applicable and generalizable.

An additional area worth exploring is identifying the most efficient E-Health communication tools for different patient groups and healthcare settings. It is vital to customize communication strategies according to preferences and technological abilities in order to enhance patient engagement and satisfaction. Furthermore, there is still much to explore regarding integrating devices and telemedicine into E-Health systems. It is essential to determine their potential to improve patient outcomes and enhance access to healthcare. Research focusing on these technologies' cost-effectiveness and scalability will guide healthcare organizations in considering their adoption.

Xu et al. (2022) assert that hospital readmissions are a concern as they lead to increased healthcare costs and highlight potential gaps in the quality of care provided to patients. E-Health systems, through telemedicine, offer features that effectively address this issue. Facilitating follow-up care enables healthcare providers to maintain communication with patients even after discharge. This ensures that patients receive instructions, medication reminders, and post-discharge support, thereby reducing the likelihood of readmission due to inadequate self-care or non-adherence to treatment. Additionally, E-Health systems can play a role in managing chronic conditions and preventing complications by providing timely reminders for follow-up appointments and medication schedules. The remote monitoring capabilities of these systems allow healthcare providers to keep track of patient's health status from a distance.

More studies have further conducted evaluations of E-Health systems in hospital settings.

Liu et al. (2017) review assesses the impact of E-Health systems on patient tracking and communication. Their findings highlight that E-Health systems significantly improve communication between patients and healthcare providers, leading to treatment progress and outcomes. Patients can easily report their health status, symptoms, and concerns, allowing for adjustments to treatment plans. An extensive review by Biancone et al. (2021) examined various E-Health communication tools used for outpatient tracking in hospital services. These tools effectively facilitated communication between patients and healthcare providers, enabling remote monitoring and support for outpatients. Secure messaging platforms allow patients to communicate with their healthcare providers, ask questions, and receive guidance, which can be particularly beneficial for managing conditions and post-operative care. Telemedicine is another E-Health communication tool that enables virtual consultations, reducing the necessity for physical visits to the hospital. This is especially valuable for patients facing barriers or limited mobility. With the help of telemedicine, healthcare professionals can perform assessments and offer guidance, resulting in better patient outcomes and fewer hospital trips.

In their study, Albahri et al. (2018) discuss the advantages of real-time E-Health tracking in hospitals. They highlighted how accessing data in time is a valuable benefit of E-Health systems, enabling healthcare professionals to make timely and informed decisions. By monitoring patient data in real time, any changes in their health or response to treatment can be promptly detected, allowing for timely interventions and adjustments to treatment plans. Additionally, real-time E-Health tracking facilitates coordination among healthcare providers. Different healthcare professionals can collaborate effectively and make well-informed decisions by accessing updated patient information. This integrated approach leads to efficient and streamlined patient care. Furthermore, patients benefit from accurate time tracking as they can actively participate in their care by accessing their health data and monitoring their progress.

In a study conducted by Iyanna et al. (2022), several challenges associated with implementing E-Health systems in hospital settings were identified. One prominent challenge is the need for an IT infrastructure capable of handling the significant amount of data generated through patient tracking and communication. Ensuring the security and privacy of this patient information is another critical concern when it comes to E-Health systems. To ensure data security, hospitals must establish robust data protection protocols and adhere to regulations regarding data privacy. Practical staff training plays a role in the successful adoption of E-Health systems. Healthcare professionals must be proficient in using E-Health tools and understanding their benefits in patient care. By receiving training, healthcare providers can maximize the potential of E-Health systems, which can lead to positive patient outcomes. In addition, resistance to change among healthcare professionals can pose a barrier when implementing E-Health systems. The shift from paper-based methods to digital systems may be met with hesitation and doubt.

Hospitals must address these concerns. Healthcare professionals must be actively involved in the implementation process to ensure smooth integration with existing workflows.

These studies highlight the advantages of E-Health systems in hospital settings regarding outpatient tracking and communication. These systems offer benefits such as reducing hospital readmission rates, improving patient outcomes, enhancing care coordination and optimizing healthcare delivery. However, it is vital to address challenges related to data privacy, security, implementation strategies, and resistance to change in the integration of E-Health systems. This study aims to contribute insights into effective implementation methods, long-term effects, and emerging trends in the field of E-Health systems.

The successful adoption of E-Health systems requires consideration of various obstacles and the development of effective strategies to tackle them. A study by Lokken et al. (2020) examined a case where a hospital successfully implemented E-Health systems to track patients. The research highlighted the role of strong leadership in driving the implementation process, gaining support from healthcare staff, and ensuring seamless integration into existing workflows. Providing training and support to healthcare professionals also proved vital in facilitating a smooth transition to using E-Health systems while maximizing their advantages. One major challenge faced while implementing E-Health systems is the need for an IT infrastructure. Hospitals must ensure that their existing technology can support the integration of E-Health systems and managing the amount of data generated by these technologies. Lokken et al. (2020) found that hospitals that invested in upgrading their IT infrastructure were better prepared to handle the demands of E-Health systems, resulting in implementation and improved patient tracking.

Another significant concern revolves around data privacy and security when it comes to utilizing E-Health systems. As the utilization of these systems increases, hospitals must prioritize safeguarding data against unauthorized access or breaches. Sivan and Zukarnain (2021) further focused on privacy and security issues. They suggested safeguarding data, including implementing robust encryption methods and strict access controls. It is vital to address these concerns to establish trust among patients regarding E-Health systems and encourage their participation. In light of focusing on patient-centered care, there has been research on how E-Health systems impact patient outcomes and treatment progress. A study conducted by (Bauer, 2018) aimed to evaluate the effectiveness of E-Health systems in a hospital setting. The results showed that hospitals that integrated E-Health systems witnessed improvements in patient outcomes, including a decrease in medical errors and better coordination among healthcare providers.

E-Health systems enhance patient outcomes by facilitating timely communication and providing healthcare teams with access to essential data. These systems allow healthcare providers to access accurate time information about patients, such as their history, diagnostic test results, and treatment plans. With this information at their fingertips, healthcare professionals can make informed decisions, leading to more accurate diagnoses and appropriate treatment interventions (Bauer, 2018). Additionally, E-Health systems promote coordination among healthcare providers by enabling a multidisciplinary approach to patient care. By consolidating information on a digital platform, professionals from different specialties can collaborate and contribute to developing an effective treatment plan. This interdisciplinary communication dramatically improves the quality of care while reducing the risk of medical errors (Bauer, 2018).

The use of patient monitoring brings numerous benefits, particularly for individuals residing in rural or distant areas. E-Health systems bridge the gap between patients and healthcare professionals, ensuring that patients receive timely medical attention and support regardless of where they are located. This approach also reduces the need for hospital visits, easing the burden on patients and healthcare facilities (Wu et al., 2022). Research literature has also examined how E-Health systems impact the roles and responsibilities of healthcare professionals within hospital settings. Bou-Karroum et al. (2020) conducted a study to explore this aspect and shed light on how adopting E-Health systems influences healthcare providers' roles. The research determined that the implementation of E-Health systems resulted in healthcare professionals experiencing a transformation in their roles. Their focus shifted towards tasks such as managing data, monitoring patients remotely and providing education to patients. The implementation of E-Health systems brings forth tools and technologies requiring healthcare professionals to acquire additional skills. For example, healthcare providers need to become proficient in utilizing E-Health platforms for accessing information and accurately interpreting data. They may also shoulder responsibilities related to remote patient monitoring and telemedicine consultations (Bou-Karroum et al., 2020).

While E-Health systems offer advantages, it is crucial for

healthcare organizations to support their staff in adapting to these changes and developing new competencies. Providing training programs and ongoing assistance becomes imperative in helping healthcare professionals fully embrace E-Health systems and unleash their potential to enhance patient care. Apart from the impact on healthcare providers, research has also explored the effects of E-Health systems on patient's attitudes and perceptions. Risling et al. (2017) conducted a study focusing on patient's acceptance and satisfaction with E-Health tracking and communication. The findings unveiled that patients who had experiences with E-Health systems were more inclined to embrace the technology actively and engage proactively in their healthcare journey. Patient acceptance and engagement are vital in successfully implementing E-Health systems. Positive patient experiences with such approaches lead to increased usage rates, as adherence ultimately results in improved treatment outcomes.

To improve acceptance, healthcare organizations must give importance to user experience and make sure that E-Health systems are easy to use, accessible, and customized according to the specific needs of each patient (Risling et al., 2017). In addition, healthcare professionals have a role in promoting the acceptance of E-Health systems among patients. By educating patients about the advantages of using E-Health technologies for tracking and communication, healthcare providers can establish trust and confidence in their patients. It is also essential to communicate about data privacy and security measures to address patient concerns and encourage them to participate actively in their healthcare (Risling et al., 2017).

Furthermore, the literature has also discussed the downsides and unintended consequences that may arise from implementing E-Health systems. McGraw, D., & Mandl, K. D. (2021) examined how these systems could potentially impact patient-provider relationships and communication in ways. While E-Health systems do offer convenience and efficiency, there are concerns that relying heavily on technology might lead to reduced face-to-face interactions, which could compromise the bond between patients and providers. Maintaining patient-provider relationships is a crucial aspect of delivering patient-centered care. E-Health systems should be seen as a complement than a replacement for traditional in-person interactions between patients and healthcare providers. Healthcare organizations need to find a balance between utilizing E-Health systems to improve care while ensuring that patients still have opportunities for personal consultations and discussions, with their healthcare providers (McGraw, D., & Mandl, K. D, 2021).

To tackle this challenge, healthcare organizations must incorporate E-Health systems in a manner that improves communication between patients and providers of impeding it. For example, healthcare providers can utilize E-Health systems to exchange health information and treatment updates with patients in between appointments, fostering continuous communication and involvement. By blending technology with care, healthcare organizations can uphold robust patient-provider relationships while capitalizing on the advantages offered by E-Health systems (Lamprinos, 2019). The literature review has emphasized the significance of implementing E-Health systems in healthcare. It discusses how these systems impact patient outcomes, aid in disease management through tracking, influence the roles of healthcare professionals, and explore patient's attitudes and perceptions. Ethical considerations and potential drawbacks of integrating E-Health systems are also addressed. By addressing these areas, healthcare organizations can overcome challenges, maximize the benefits of E-Health systems and ultimately improve care and healthcare delivery. This study aims to contribute to this field by examining how to integrate E-Health systems into hospital services and offering valuable insights into successful implementation strategies.

The literature review highlights how E-Health systems play a role in transforming hospital services for outpatient tracking and communication. These systems have proven to enhance outcomes, improve care coordination, and increase patient engagement. However, there are still some challenges that need to be addressed, such as data privacy, security concerns, and implementation barriers. To fully leverage the benefits of E-Health systems, it is necessary to address these challenges. As technology continues to evolve, further research is needed to explore emerging trends like AI integration, wearable devices, and telemedicine, ensuring that healthcare delivery remains patient-centric and efficient. The aim of this study is to fill the existing gaps in the literature by providing insights into effectively integrating E-Health systems into hospital services for outpatient tracking and communication.

SUMMARY

The review of existing literature has highlighted significant themes related to how E-Health systems are used in hospitals for tracking and communication with outpatient services. These systems have proven to be highly beneficial in improving patient outcomes, coordinating care, effectively engaging patients in their healthcare, and optimizing the delivery of healthcare services. By using E-Health systems for accurate time tracking and communication, healthcare providers can intervene promptly and create care plans. Patients also benefit from these systems as they empower them with knowledge about their conditions and help them adhere to treatment plans effectively. Furthermore, integrating intelligent wearable devices and telemedicine into E-Health systems can potentially transform patient care and treatment planning.

However, despite the results shown in the literature, some gaps still need attention. Certain studies have identified challenges related to data privacy, security concerns, and the successful implementation of E-Health systems within hospital settings. Additionally, further research is required to evaluate the long-term effects of these systems on patient health outcomes and overall healthcare results. Conducting studies focusing on strategies and best practices for successfully implementing E-Health systems would enhance our understanding of this topic.

THE PRESENT STUDY

The present study aims to fill the identified gap in the literature by providing valuable insights into the effective integration of E-Health systems in hospital services for outpatient tracking and communication. The research has addressed the challenges related to data privacy and security concerns by implementing robust data protection measures to safeguard patient information (Maksimović & Vujović, 2017). Additionally, the study has investigated the strategies and best practices for successful E-Health system implementation in hospital settings, with a focus on strong leadership, staff involvement, and ongoing support and training.

Furthermore, the study has evaluated the long-term effects of E-Health systems on patient health and healthcare outcomes. By conducting a qualitative study, the research has assessed the sustained impact of E-Health tracking and communication on patient engagement, treatment adherence, and overall healthcare quality.

To explore emerging trends, the study has investigated the integration of artificial intelligence in E-Health systems for predictive analytics and personalized treatment planning. Moreover, the research has examined the potential benefits of wearable devices and telemedicine in enhancing remote patient tracking and monitoring, particularly for patients in rural or remote areas. The gaps found in research, such as the need for effective strategies to tackle challenges in implementing E-Health systems, understanding their impact on patient outcomes, and addressing ethical considerations, will guide the methods discussed in Chapter 3. The study takes two approaches: conducting qualitative interviews with healthcare professionals and analyzing quantitative data from patient records. This combination of methods has allowed for an exploration of the implementation process, patient outcomes, and ethical implications. The findings have provided insights to fill the existing gaps in the literature and expand existing knowledge in integrating E-Health systems into hospital services.

SECTION 3: RESEARCH METHODOLOGY

ROLE OF THE RESEARCHER RESEARCH METHODOLOGY

In the process of conducting this research, practical methodologies and established algorithms were drawn from methodological literature to guide the transformation of data sets into reliable findings (Qandeel, 2022). The researcher's transition into a pivotal instrument for comprehending and interpreting qualitative information was a key aspect of this endeavor (Qandeel, 2022). Data from previous studies were utilized through a comprehensive literature review, which aided in formulating a clear research direction. After a thorough understanding of the study context was achieved, data collection techniques were chosen, with due consideration of findings from analogous research endeavors (Mitnik, 2020).

According to Mohajan (2018), the role of the researcher encompassed the selection and recruitment of participants who aligned with the predefined inclusion criteria of the study. This involved securing informed consent from participants and taking measures to safeguard their privacy and maintain confidentiality. Data quality assurance was an integral responsibility, involving meticulous scrutiny for errors, inconsistencies, and missing data. Efforts were directed toward guaranteeing the completeness and impartiality of the collected data. Effective management and organization of the amassed data were essential components, ensuring its secure storage and facilitating streamlined access for subsequent analysis (Cypress, 2018).

DISCUSSION ON THE POPULATION AND SAMPLING

STUDY POPULATION

In typical research, the population was defined as the group capable of fulfilling the study's objectives (Campbell et al., 2020). This study's population consisted of individuals employed within a healthcare facility utilizing the E-Health system. The scope of such facilities often extends widely, operating on a global scale. Given the challenges posed by sampling from numerous sources, a more efficient approach was to concentrate on a specific healthcare facility. Consequently, the study focused on individuals working at a healthcare facility employing the E-Health system.

According to Thomas (2016), limiting the study participants to a specific healthcare facility was a deliberate choice in alignment with the study's specific focus. By confining the research to this facility, the investigation adopted a more targeted and manageable approach to data collection, facilitating the exploration of the research inquiries effectively. This strategic decision streamlined the data collection process and allowed for a deeper understanding of how the E-Health system was integrated and experienced within the chosen healthcare facility.

STUDY SAMPLE

The researcher aimed to select a sample of approximately 20 participants from the healthcare facility. The participants included employees with direct experience and involvement in the E-Health system, such as administrators, nurses, doctors, and support staff. Various roles and responsibilities within the chosen facility were considered to ensure a comprehensive array of viewpoints. The participants' age ranges and duration of service reflected the diverse composition of the workforce within the specific facility under study.

ELIGIBLE PARTICIPANTS

Eligibility requirements determine the usefulness of individuals as subjects in the study (Mohajan, 2018). Participants with experience in the E-Health system were deemed relevant due to their potential to offer valuable insights into the system's effectiveness. According to Campbell et al. (2020), specific inclusion criteria must be met for a person to be eligible, while exclusion criteria determine who cannot participate (Kegler et al., 2019). For this research study, eligible participants were employees of Golden Years Care who met the following criteria:

a) Understanding the facility's E-Health systems was essential. Participants needed to possess a solid comprehension of the E-Health systems utilized within the facility.

b) The facility encompassed various roles and responsibilities, including administrators, nurses, doctors, and support staff. This diverse representation ensured a comprehensive perspective on the E-Health system's implementation and functionality.

c) Length of service at the facility ensured a sufficient understanding of the E-Health system's implementation and operation. Participants were required to have a tenure substantial enough to offer insights based on experience with the system over time.

d) Participants were expected to contribute insights into the effectiveness or ineffectiveness of E-Health. Their perspectives were crucial in evaluating the impact of the system on their roles and the overall healthcare processes.

By adhering to these eligibility criteria, the study aimed to gather comprehensive insights into the experiences and perceptions of employees at Golden Years Care regarding the E-Health system. These criteria ensured that the selected participants possessed the knowledge and experience necessary to contribute valuable information to the research, enhancing the study's overall rigor and effectiveness.

DATA SECURITY AND PARTICIPANT CONFIDENTIALITY

In the research process, we were highly conscious of protecting the identities and confidentiality of all participants, including staff involved in overseeing patient records. We took several measures to ensure their privacy:

Anonymity: We assigned pseudonyms to all participants in our study. This conceals their true identities and allows us to present their responses without any risk of identification.

Confidentiality: We stored all collected data securely, ensuring it was only accessible to the research team. This protected sensitive information from being disclosed inadvertently.

Informed Consent: Participants were informed of the study's purpose and provided explicit consent for their involvement. They knew their participation was voluntary, and they could withdraw anytime.

Data Security: Electronic data was encrypted and password-protected, and hard copies of any documents were securely stored.

These measures collectively aimed to safeguard the identities and information of all participants, maintaining the highest ethical standards throughout the research.

REASONS FOR ELIGIBILITY

Relevant knowledge: Participants with experience using E-Health systems would likely possess the necessary insights and skills for the study.

Quality engagement: Participants familiar with E-Health systems demonstrated higher engagement and willingness to participate in the study. This increased engagement contributed to improved recruitment and reduced dropout rates, ultimately leading to a more successful study.

POPULATION SAMPLING PROCESS

Sampling methods are another name for the varied selection techniques. According to Sullivan et al. (2019), sampling is choosing a representative sample of a target population. An example should be expected because it should have a size sufficient for a compelling study and adequate to represent the entire population (Ames et al., 2019). It is often necessary to choose only a portion of the target group for study participation because there are frequently too many (Knechel, 2019).

The researcher first defined the target population as individuals with prior experience using the E-Health system at the Golden Years Care facility—the second step aimed to purposively select participants from a list of individuals meeting the inclusion criteria. The facility's management provided the list of potential participants. In the third step, the sample size of 20 participants was determined. This size was chosen based on research objectives, data saturation, and feasibility. The decision to include 20 participants was made to ensure in-depth insights into qualitative research while prioritizing the richness of data over a larger sample size. This approach aligned well with the study's aims, chosen methodology, and available resources, guaranteeing validity and data saturation within a manageable timeframe.

The researcher then opted for a sampling technique, choosing to use purposive sampling for this qualitative research. Participants were selected purposefully based on their expertise and experience in the E-Healthcare field. This approach ensured that the insights provided by the selected participants would closely align with the study's focus on challenges related to the utilization of the E-Health system.

Lastly, the researcher recruited and selected participants using a fair, transparent, and ethical process. Clear criteria were established to determine eligibility for participation. Informed consent was obtained from all participants, ensuring they understood the nature of the study and their voluntary involvement. Confidentiality measures were put in place to safeguard participants' privacy. Participation was entirely voluntary, and participants were assured that their decision to participate or not would not affect their relationship with the facility. Ethical approval was obtained to ensure the research adhered to ethical standards.

Moreover, the researcher promoted equal opportunity by ensuring that potential participants were approached and selected without bias or discrimination.

STUDY SAMPLES AND METHODS FOR DETERMINING THE SAMPLES

Determining an appropriate sample size was a critical aspect of the research design, as it directly impacted the study's validity and the generalizability of its findings. In the case of the study, which aimed to investigate the underutilization of E-Health systems within the healthcare facility, the selection of a sample size of 20 participants warranted a more comprehensive rationale.

Rationale for Sample Size

The selected sample size of 20 participants was strategically chosen to encompass a diverse range of roles within the healthcare facility. This inclusivity ensured that the study captured insights from various perspectives and positions, enhancing the richness and depth of the data collected. Given the limitations in terms of time and resources, a larger sample size might not have been feasible (Lakens, 2022). A sample size of 20 struck a balance between obtaining comprehensive data and ensuring the study's practicability and manageability within the designated timeframe.

With a sample size of 20 participants, the study could effectively capture a spectrum of experiences, opinions, and challenges related to E-Health system utilization. This variability was crucial for generating insights that accurately represented the facility's staff as a whole.

A sample size of 20 was statistically robust, especially for qualitative research and case studies. It allowed for identifying patterns, themes, and trends in the data, facilitating the achievement of research objectives (Lakens, 2022). The sample size of 20 was based on participants who met the predefined inclusion criteria, ensuring that only individuals with

Relevant experience and knowledge of the utilization of the E-Health system were included. This focused approach enhanced the study's validity and relevance to the research question.

Population Coverage

It is essential to clarify that while a sample size of 20 participants did cover approximately 60% of the facility's staff, this percentage alone did not substantiate the sample size selection (Lakens, 2022). Instead, the selection was primarily driven by the above mentioned factors: representing diverse roles, accommodating resource constraints, capturing data variability, and maintaining statistical rigor. In retrospect, the chosen sample size of 20 participants for this study was justified by its capacity to provide comprehensive insights into the underutilization of E-Health systems within the healthcare facility. The rationale considered factors such as population representation, resource limitations, data variability, and statistical rigor, ensuring that the study's findings were meaningful and applicable to the broader context of the facility's staff.

DETAILED DESCRIPTIONS

RECRUITING

All selected participants for this study received an announcement about the research and were presented with an acceptance form to participate. The recruitment strategy involved informing potential participants about the study and enticing those who met the criteria for the E-Health system's research to volunteer. In addition to the initial announcement and acceptance form, the researcher followed up with potential participants through various channels such as email, phone calls, or in-person communication to ensure maximum participation. In situations where the initial recruitment strategy required more participants, alternative approaches, such as targeted outreach and referrals from existing participants were considered to provide an adequate sample size and collaboration with relevant departments or staff members.

SELECTION

The exclusion method eliminated those with little experience in the E-Health system, leaving only the most qualified subjects for the study (Stoll et al., 2019). The participant selection method involved selecting individuals randomly from the population of those who met the inclusion criteria. The selection's randomness helped reduce bias in the sample by ensuring that every individual in the population had an equal chance of being included.

PROCEDURES FOR ASSIGNING TO GROUPS

The selection process successfully influenced the organization of the research subjects.

According to Calvillo-Arbizu et al. (2019), grouping participants was crucial as group interviews played a vital role in gathering data for the study. Participants were randomly assigned to different groups to enable researchers to control variables that could impact the study's outcomes (Acharya et al., 2019). This approach ensured that any differences observed between the groups were attributed to the intervention under study rather than other factors, as highlighted by Acharya et al. (2019). In addition to the interview discussions, each subject was randomly allocated to one of the four groups comprising five participants. The researcher provided participants with the option to choose their preferred group while also randomly assigning those participants who did not express a preference. This balanced approach ensured that the groups were equitable concerning other factors, such as employee relationships, which could have influenced the study's outcomes.

GAINING ACCESS TO THE SAMPLE

A letter requesting access permission was sent to the facility in conjunction with the invitation request to the identified staff members at the facility. The sample consisted of individuals who were on-site at the facility for the entire five-hour workday, from 8 a.m. to 1 p.m. To accommodate participants, the interview discussions were scheduled during business hours. A week before each interview, informing the facility manager of the upcoming interview session was deemed essential.

THE ACTUAL PARTICIPANTS

The actual participants in this study consisted of 20 employees from Golden Years Care facility who had knowledge and proficiency with the E-Health system. Most participants were working nurses, considering their direct involvement in patient care and their role in utilizing the E-Health system. It is important to note that the participants were over the age of 20 and had post-high school education, as this demographic was likely to possess the necessary skills and experience to provide valuable insights into the system's implementation and effectiveness (Lakens, 2022). Other relevant roles within the facility, such as administrators or support staff, were also included to gather diverse perspectives on the E-Health system's utilization and impact.

SUMMARY

The participants in this study were selected from employees at the Golden Years Healthcare facility who had experience with the E-Health system. The sampling process involved defining the target population, identifying the sampling frame, determining the sample size, choosing a sampling technique, and engaging in recruiting and selecting participants. A random sample of 20 participants was selected to participate in the study. The recruitment strategy involved informing potential participants about the study and inviting those who met the criteria for the E-Health system research to volunteer. The selection process ensured that only experienced participants were included in the study. Finally, participants were assigned to different groups through a random process, ensuring that the groups were balanced with other factors that could affect the study's outcome.

DATA COLLECTION AND ANALYSIS

DATA COLLECTION

Data for this study was collected through one-on-one semi-structured interviews with staff members who had experience using the E-Health system. The interview discussions were guided by open-ended questions, allowing participants to freely express their experiences, opinions, and challenges related to the E-Health system. The semi-structured format ensured interview consistency, allowing participants to elaborate on their unique perspectives.

DATA ANALYSIS

The analysis of the collected data was a critical step in ensuring the validity and reliability of the study's findings. This study employed a mixed-methods approach, combining qualitative and quantitative analysis methods, to comprehensively address the research questions and achieve triangulation of interview data.

Qualitative Analysis

Narrative and Thematic Analysis: The qualitative data collected through semi-structured interviews underwent narrative and thematic analysis. Narrative analysis involved creating a coherent and detailed account of each participant's experiences, perceptions, and viewpoints. This method provided a rich description of individual perspectives, allowing for a deeper understanding of the participants' unique experiences with the E-Health system. Thematic analysis, however, involved identifying common patterns, themes, and trends that emerged across the participants' narratives. In line with Kiger and Varpio (2020) guidelines, this coding and theme development process enabled the extraction of meaningful insights related to the effectiveness and ineffectiveness of the E-Health system.

Coding Process

The qualitative data was transcribed verbatim and subjected to open coding, where the data was broken down into meaningful segments. This initial coding phase allowed the identification of various concepts, issues, and categories in the data. Through axial coding, relationships between different codes were established, facilitating the development of overarching themes. These themes were refined through selective coding, creating a comprehensive thematic framework that aligned with the research questions.

Triangulation and Data Triangulation

The study employed triangulation at both the data and analysis levels to enhance the credibility and rigor of the findings. Data triangulation involves the use of multiple data sources, such as interviews, documents, and observations, to validate and corroborate the findings. In this study, qualitative interviews were triangulated with quantitative survey data from the facility's records, ensuring a comprehensive exploration of the E-Health system's effectiveness.

Quantitative Analysis

Quantitative analysis involved statistical techniques to analyze survey data collected from the facility's records. Descriptive statistics provided an overview of the utilization patterns, trends, and frequencies related to the E-Health system (Mishra et al., 2019). Quantitative data were used to complement qualitative insights, enriching the study's findings by providing numerical context to qualitative narratives.

Triangulation of Qualitative and Quantitative Data

The qualitative and quantitative data were integrated through data triangulation. This process involved comparing and contrasting findings from both data sources to identify areas of convergence and divergence. Triangulation enhanced the robustness of the findings, as consistent patterns identified through different methods lent more credibility to the research outcomes (Moon, 2019).

References to Leading Authorities

The analysis approach was drawn from leading authorities in qualitative research and case study methodologies. Grounded theory (1968), as outlined by Glaser and Strauss (1968), guided the coding and thematic analysis process. A comprehensive framework for conducting case studies informed the study's overall design, data collection, and analysis strategies. The data analysis process combined narrative and thematic analysis for qualitative data and employed descriptive statistical techniques for quantitative data. Triangulation, both in terms of data sources and analysis methods, ensured a comprehensive exploration of the research questions, contributing to the validity and credibility of the study's findings.

ASSUMPTIONS, LIMITATIONS, DELIMITATIONS

ASSUMPTIONS

Participant Honesty: One critical assumption in this study was that participants would provide honest and accurate responses during the interviews. Efforts were made to establish a safe and confidential environment for sharing experiences. However, it was acknowledged that there might be variations in participants' willingness to fully disclose their perceptions and experiences with the E-Health system, impacting the reliability and validity of the data collected. The assumption of participant honesty was considered vital to gain a comprehensive and accurate understanding of the factors influencing the effectiveness and ineffectiveness of the E-Health system at the healthcare facility.

Representativeness of Sample: Another assumption made was that the selected sample of participants reasonably represented the target population of healthcare professionals using the E-Health system at the facility. This assumption was crucial to ensure the study's findings could be generalized to similar healthcare settings. While efforts were made to select participants based on their previous use of the E-Health system, it was recognized that different healthcare professionals' experiences and perspectives could exist.

Participant Comprehension: It was assumed that participants comprehended the interview questions and provided relevant and meaningful responses. This assumption was essential to ensure the collected data aligned with the research questions and objectives. To address this assumption, the researcher validated the interview questions before conducting interviews and provided clear instructions to ensure participant understanding.

Absence of Response Bias: The assumption of the absence of response bias was maintained to ensure that participants did not provide socially desirable responses or withhold information due to fear of judgment. The researcher emphasized confidentiality and anonymity to mitigate response bias and maintained a non-judgmental stance during interviews. Despite these efforts, the possibility of response bias was acknowledged, and the researcher remained cautious during data analysis and interpretation.

Absence of External Factors: The assumption was that no

significant external factors or events during the data collection period could substantially impact participants' experiences with the E-Health system. Recognizing that external factors could influence participants' perceptions and introduce confounding variables, the researcher contextualized the study findings within the specific data collection timeframe.

These assumptions were considered integral to conducting a meaningful and valid study. Acknowledging these assumptions enabled the researcher to address potential limitations transparently and enhance the credibility and applicability of the research findings.

LIMITATIONS

Several limitations were recognized that could influence the interpretation of the study's findings. Interviews conducted during regular business hours may have constrained participants due to time limitations imposed by their work responsibilities. The urgency of the deadline might have curtailed participants' ability to express their experiences comprehensively. The bustling environment of the healthcare facility could have added noise and disturbances, possibly hampering participants' concentration and responses during interviews.

Another potential limitation pertains to social desirability bias in participant responses. Participants might have hesitated to voice discontent with the E-Health system due to concerns about how their colleagues or supervisors might react. To mitigate this, the interviewer underscored the confidentiality and anonymity of the feedback.

Moreover, the researcher's biases and presumptions could have impacted the findings, underscoring the need for an objective and neutral stance during interviews. As emphasized by Mohajan (2018), acknowledging limitations is crucial for thoroughly assessing study findings. Despite these limitations, the study offers valuable insights into staff members' utilization of the E-Health system within a healthcare context, along with recommendations for enhancing its usability and effectiveness.

Several limitations were encountered during this study:

Generalizability: The findings were context-specific centered around the studied healthcare facility and its unique E-Health system. Therefore, the results might not extend seamlessly to other healthcare settings with distinct contexts, infrastructure, or user demographics (Prabhu, 2020).

Sample size: Although efforts were made to ensure diversity within the sample, the study's sample size remained relatively small. Consequently, the captured perspectives and experiences may not encapsulate the full spectrum of views concerning the E-Health system.

Subjectivity: Given the qualitative nature of the study, a degree of subjectivity was inherent in the data analysis process. Despite striving for objectivity, the researcher's biases and preconceptions could have influenced the interpretation of interview responses and the identification of themes.

Recall bias: Participants' accounts of their interactions with the E-Health system were susceptible to recall bias, as they relied on memory during the interview process. This bias may have affected the accuracy and comprehensiveness of the collected data.

DELIMITATIONS

Geographic Boundary: The study was limited to the Golden Years Care facility located in a specific geographical area. The findings may not be generalizable to other healthcare facilities in different regions due to organizational practices, infrastructure, and technology adoption variations.

Sample Demographics: The study included healthcare professionals, such as doctors, nurses, and administrative staff, who had experience using the E-Health system at the Golden Years Care facility. The sample demographics may not have represented the entire healthcare workforce, and the findings may not have applied to healthcare professionals with different backgrounds or experiences.

Time Frame: The data collection for this study was conducted within a specific time frame, and any changes in the E-Health system or organizational practices beyond this period may not have been captured. As technology and organizational processes evolve, the relevance of the findings may diminish over time.

Language: The interviews were conducted in a specific language that may have limited the inclusion of non-English-speaking healthcare professionals, potentially affecting the diversity of perspectives represented in the study.

Nature of the Facility: The study focused on a single healthcare facility with unique characteristics, culture, and resources. The findings may not have been transferable to different types of healthcare organizations, such as large hospitals or smaller clinics, with distinct operational contexts.

SECTION 4: RESULTS, DISCUSSIONS AND IMPLICATIONS

RESULTS

The results of this study provide valuable insights into the underutilization of E-Health services in healthcare practices and the factors contributing to employee resistance to organizational change. Through a thorough analysis of data collected from healthcare professionals, several key findings emerged, shedding light on the root causes of these challenges and potential strategies to address them.

UNDERUTILIZATION OF E-HEALTH SERVICES IN HEALTHCARE PRACTICES

The study found that the underutilization of E-Health services in healthcare practices is primarily driven by two main factors: inadequate training and technical support and concerns about data privacy and security. Healthcare professionals lacked confidence in using the E-Health system due to insufficient training and support during implementation (Risling et al., 2017). Many reported that they were not adequately trained on the system's functionalities, leading to confusion and hesitancy in utilizing its full potential. Data privacy and security concerns emerged as significant barriers to E-Health system adoption. Healthcare professionals expressed apprehensions about the confidentiality of patient information and potential data breaches (Maksimović & Vujović, 2017). These concerns hindered their willingness to fully embrace the system and share sensitive patient data, limiting its effectiveness in delivering comprehensive and coordinated patient care.

EMPLOYEE RESISTANCE TO ORGANIZATIONAL CHANGE IN HEALTHCARE SETTINGS

The study also explored employee resistance to organizational change in healthcare settings, particularly during the implementation of E-Health systems. The findings revealed that employee resistance is influenced by factors such as fear of job insecurity, lack of involvement in decision-making processes, and resistance to changes in daily work routines. Healthcare professionals expressed challenges in adapting to new technologies and processes, leading to resistance and reluctance to embrace organizational changes. Organizational culture was identified as a significant factor influencing employee resistance to change. Healthcare organizations with hierarchical and traditional cultures faced more considerable opposition, as employees perceived a lack of openness to feedback and a rigid approach to change. In contrast, organizations with more inclusive and adaptive cultures reported lower levels of employee resistance, as employees felt more empowered and supported during the change process.

DISCUSSIONS

UNDERUTILIZATION OF E-HEALTH SERVICES

The study's findings revealed that the underutilization of E-Health services in healthcare practices is a multi-faceted issue with significant implications for patient care and organizational efficiency. Inadequate training and technical support emerged as prominent barriers to system utilization. Healthcare professionals lacked confidence in using the E-Health system due to insufficient training during implementation. This finding suggests that healthcare organizations must prioritize comprehensive training programs to ensure that staff members can effectively utilize the system's functionalities. Moreover, data privacy and security concerns were identified as key factors contributing to underutilization (Bauer, 2018). Healthcare professionals expressed apprehensions about the confidentiality of patient information and potential data breaches. Addressing these concerns is essential to building trust and encouraging healthcare professionals to share sensitive patient data through the E-Health system. Robust data privacy and security measures, such as encryption protocols and access controls, must be implemented to alleviate these concerns.

EMPLOYEE RESISTANCE TO ORGANIZATIONAL CHANGE

The study's exploration of employee resistance to organizational change shed light on the challenges healthcare organizations face when introducing E-Health systems. Fear of job insecurity, lack of involvement in decision-making processes, and resistance to changes in daily work routines were identified as factors influencing resistance. These findings underscore the importance of involving employees in the change process and fostering a culture of open communication. Organizational culture emerged as a significant factor influencing employee resistance. Hierarchical and traditional cultures were associated with higher resistance levels, while inclusive and adaptive cultures reported lower resistance levels. Healthcare leaders must strive to create an organizational culture that embraces change as an opportunity for growth and empowers employees to adapt to new technologies and processes (Bauer, 2018).

PRACTICAL IMPLICATIONS FOR HEALTHCARE ORGANIZATIONS

The discussions highlight the practical implications of the study's findings for healthcare organizations. Addressing the challenges of E-Health system underutilization and employee resistance to organizational change requires a strategic and holistic approach. Healthcare leaders must recognize the importance of investing in training and support to maximize the E-Health system's potential and improve patient care outcomes. Creating a culture of open communication and employee involvement is essential to overcome resistance to organizational change (Errida & Lotfi, 2021). Healthcare organizations can foster a sense of ownership and commitment to change initiatives by actively engaging employees in the change process and valuing their input. The study's findings also emphasize the significance of data privacy and security in building trust among healthcare professionals. Healthcare organizations must prioritize data protection measures to ensure patient information is secure, thereby encouraging greater data sharing and utilization through the E-Health system.

RELATIONSHIP OF FINDINGS

The Research Questions

The findings of this study directly address the research questions posed in the study. The investigation into the underutilization of E-Health services and employee resistance to organizational change yielded insightful responses that shed light on the underlying factors contributing to these challenges. Specifically, the study revealed that inadequate training, technical support, and data privacy and security concerns contribute to E-Health system underutilization. Similarly, employee resistance is influenced by fear of job insecurity, lack of involvement in decision-making, and resistance to changes in daily routines.

The Research Framework

The study's findings harmonize closely with the conceptual framework rooted in the Technology Acceptance Model (TAM), a well-regarded theory for understanding technology adoption. The model's core constructs, including perceived ease of use and perceived usefulness, strongly resonate with the identified challenges in E-Health system adoption. Participants' responses aptly correspond to the model's categories of technology users, displaying varying degrees of readiness to accept and integrate the E-Health system into their practices (Wahyuni, 2017). The interplay between the model's elements, such as user perceptions, external variables, and behavioral intentions, vividly mirrors the study's discoveries concerning training effectiveness, data security concerns, organizational cultural impact, and employee attitudes toward change.

Anticipated Themes

The study's findings correspond with the anticipated themes, confirming the significance of training, data security, and organizational culture in influencing E-Health system utilization and employee resistance to change. These findings support the importance of the anticipated themes while also uncovering unanticipated insights, such as the nuanced role of data privacy concerns in hindering E-Health system adoption. This emphasizes the complexity of challenges and the need for a comprehensive approach.

The Literature

The study's findings contribute to the existing literature by corroborating and expanding upon previous research. The challenges of inadequate training and technical support identified in the study resonate with literature highlighting the importance of user training in technology adoption. Similarly, the findings regarding data privacy concerns align with literature discussing barriers to digital transformation in healthcare. The link between organizational culture and employee resistance supports literature on change management and its emphasis on fostering adaptable cultures.

However, the study also reveals some nuances that diverge from the literature. The specific interplay between organizational culture and employee resistance is a notable departure from the generalized discussions in the literature. This suggests that the impact of organizational culture on employee attitudes toward change might be more intricate than previously explored. The findings of this study establish a strong connection to the research questions, the research framework, anticipated themes, and the existing literature. The study affirms established ideas and introduces novel insights that enrich the understanding of E-Health system underutilization and employee resistance in healthcare settings.

IMPLICATIONS AND RECOMMENDATIONS FOR FUTURE RESEARCH

The findings of this study have significant implications for healthcare organizations seeking to optimize E-Health system utilization and overcome employee resistance to organizational change. The discussions revealed several critical areas for consideration and provided insights into potential strategies for improvement. This section will discuss the study's findings' implications and provide future research recommendations.

IMPLICATIONS

Training and Support: The study highlighted the importance of comprehensive training and technical support for healthcare professionals to utilize the E-Health system effectively.

Healthcare organizations must recognize the significance of ongoing training programs that provide hands-on experiences and address user concerns (Manzini et al., 2020). Implementing robust training and support initiatives will empower healthcare professionals to maximize the system's potential and improve patient care outcomes.

Data Privacy and Security: Data privacy and security concerns emerged as significant barriers to E-Health system utilization. McGraw, D., & Mandl, K. D. (2021) recommend that healthcare organizations prioritize data protection measures to build trust among healthcare professionals and patients. Strengthening data governance policies, implementing encryption protocols, and adopting access controls will enhance data security and encourage greater data sharing and utilization.

Employee Involvement and Communication: Employee resistance to organizational change can be mitigated by actively involving healthcare professionals in decision-making processes and fostering open communication channels (Potnuru et al., 2023). Healthcare leaders must recognize the value of employee feedback and input and communicate the rationale behind change initiatives. By involving employees in the change process, healthcare organizations can create a sense of ownership and commitment to organizational goals.

Organizational Culture: The study highlighted the role of corporate culture in influencing employee resistance to change. Healthcare organizations must strive to cultivate a positive, adaptable culture that embraces innovation and continuous improvement. Recognizing and rewarding employee contributions, providing opportunities for skill development, and promoting a learning culture will encourage employees to embrace change positively (Moloney et al., 2020).

RECOMMENDATIONS FOR FUTURE RESEARCH

Long-Term Impacts: Future research could explore the long-term impacts of E-Health system utilization on patient care outcomes and organizational efficiency. This could include evaluating patient satisfaction, healthcare provider productivity, and cost savings achieved through the ongoing use of E-Health services. Longitudinal studies could provide valuable insights into the sustained effects of E-Health system utilization over time (Wang et al., 2021).

Comparative Studies: Conducting comparative studies between healthcare organizations that have successfully optimized E-Health system utilization and those facing challenges could offer valuable insights. Identifying best practices and success factors could inform the development of targeted interventions to effectively address underutilization and resistance to change.

User Experience and Satisfaction: According to Anshari et al. (2021), investigating healthcare professionals' experiences and satisfaction with the E-Health system could provide valuable feedback for system improvement. Understanding user preferences, pain points, and suggestions for enhancement will enable healthcare organizations to tailor the system to meet user needs effectively.

Implementation Strategies: Research exploring different implementation strategies for E-Health systems in healthcare organizations could shed light on the most effective approaches to foster system adoption and utilization. Comparative studies of varying implementation methodologies, such as phased rollouts versus full-scale implementations, could offer valuable insights into the factors influencing successful performance.

Impact on Healthcare Outcomes: Future research could assess the effects of E-Health system utilization on specific healthcare outcomes, such as reduced hospital readmission rates, improved chronic disease management, and enhanced care coordination. Understanding how E-Health services contribute to improved patient care and products will strengthen the evidence base for their value in healthcare practices (Bauer, 2018).

Cultural Change Initiatives: Further research on strategies to foster cultural change within healthcare organizations could address employee resistance to organizational change. Exploring successful cultural change initiatives and leadership practices could inform healthcare leaders on effective strategies to create a culture that embraces innovation and change.

Cost-Benefit Analysis: Conducting cost-benefit analyses of E-Health system implementation could provide insights into the financial implications of investment in these technologies.

Understanding the potential cost savings and return on investment will help healthcare organizations make informed decisions about adopting and utilizing E-Health services (Yusif et al., 2017).

The implications of this study emphasize the importance of comprehensive training, data privacy and security, employee involvement, and organizational culture in optimizing E-Health system utilization. Addressing these challenges requires a strategic and holistic approach from healthcare organizations. Future research can build on these findings by exploring long-term impacts, conducting comparative studies, assessing user experience, investigating implementation strategies, evaluating healthcare outcomes, analyzing cultural change initiatives, and conducting cost-benefit analyses. By addressing these areas, healthcare organizations can unlock the full potential of E-Health services and drive positive patient care outcomes and organizational efficiency.

Reliability and Validity

The reliability and validity of research findings were meticulously upheld throughout the conducted study, ensuring the credibility and robustness of its outcomes. To enhance reliability, a comprehensive approach was taken:

Prolonged Engagement: Immersion within the E-Healthcare facility enabled an in-depth understanding of the context and participants, fostering accuracy and trustworthiness in data collection.

Triangulation: Findings were validated through diverse data sources, including interviews with healthcare professionals, cross-referencing with pertinent documents, and potential integration of direct observations.

Member Checking: Participants were engaged in member checking, corroborating the precision of researcher interpretations and confirming the accurate reflection of their viewpoints.

Peer Debriefing: Insights were shared with peers and mentors, stimulating discussions on biases, refining interpretations, and bolstering the study's credibility.

The pursuit of validity encompassed several key dimensions

Credibility: Building rapport, conducting in-depth interviews, and thoroughly immersing in the research setting established credibility and captured rich and nuanced data.

Transferability: Transparently documented research context, participant selection, and data collection methods facilitated the assessment of findings' applicability to similar contexts.

Dependability: Methodical documentation encompassed the research process, bolstering dependability through a traceable decision-making trail.

Confirmability: Reflexivity and potential biases were acknowledged and managed transparently, with reflexive journaling unveiling the researcher's perspectives and influences. To address biases, bracketing techniques were adroitly employed:

Reflexive Journaling: Maintaining a reflexive journal throughout the study documented personal biases, fostering awareness and minimizing their impact on data and analysis.

Peer Debriefing: Consultation with peers and mentors provided an external perspective, rectifying any unintentional biases that could have influenced the research.

Member Checking: Feedback from participants during

member checking aided in identifying potential biases in analysis, ensuring their voices remained authentically represented.

Reliability and validity were upheld through prolonged engagement, triangulation, member checking, and peer debriefing. The study maintained credibility, transferability, dependability, and confirmability to enhance validity. Employed bracketing techniques, comprising reflexive journaling, peer debriefing, and member checking, adeptly managed potential biases, preserving the study's objectivity. The cumulative impact of these rigorous methodologies instilled confidence in the study's trustworthiness and the caliber of its findings.

SUMMARY AND STUDY CONCLUSION

SUMMARY

This study explored the underutilization of E-Health systems in healthcare practices and its impact on patient care outcomes and organizational efficiency. A thorough review of the existing literature and primary research identified key challenges and barriers that hinder the complete adoption and utilization of E-Health systems in healthcare facilities.

The study has highlighted the significance of comprehensive training and technical support for healthcare professionals to utilize E-Health systems effectively. Ongoing training programs that address user concerns and provide hands-on experiences have empowered healthcare professionals to maximize the system's potential and improve patient care outcomes. Data privacy and security concerns emerged as crucial factors affecting system utilization. Strengthening data protection measures, implementing encryption protocols, and adopting access controls are essential to enhancing data security and encouraging greater data sharing and utilization.

Furthermore, the study has uncovered the importance of

employee involvement and communication in mitigating resistance to organizational change. Actively involving healthcare professionals in decision-making and fostering open communication channels creates a sense of ownership and commitment to organizational goals. Moreover, the study has emphasized the role of organizational culture in influencing employee resistance to change. A positive and adaptable culture that embraces innovation and continuous improvement can foster positive attitudes toward change and innovation.

The implications of this study are significant and relevant to the healthcare industry. By addressing the identified challenges and implementing the proposed strategies, healthcare organizations can optimize E-Health system utilization, improving patient care experiences and organizational effectiveness. E-Health systems' successful adoption and utilization require a multifaceted approach and collaborative efforts among healthcare providers, administrators, and other stakeholders to embrace change and overcome barriers.

As a researcher, I believe that this study can serve as a stepping stone for future research in this field. Further studies can build upon these findings to explore long-term impacts, conduct comparative analyses, assess user experiences, evaluate implementation strategies, explore cultural change initiatives, and conduct cost-benefit studies. Continuous research and innovation will advance healthcare services and ultimately improve patient care and organizational effectiveness in the ever-evolving healthcare landscape.

CONCLUSION

This study has delved into the underutilization of E-Health systems in healthcare practices and its impact on patient care outcomes and organizational efficiency. Through thoroughly exploring the literature and primary research, we have identified key challenges and barriers that hinder the complete adoption and utilization of E-Health systems in healthcare facilities. The findings emphasize the significance of comprehensive training and technical support for healthcare professionals to utilize E-Health systems effectively. Ongoing training programs that address user concerns and provide hands-on experiences empower healthcare professionals to maximize the system's potential and improve patient care outcomes.

Data privacy and security concerns emerged as crucial factors affecting system utilization. Strengthening data protection measures, implementing encryption protocols, and adopting access controls are essential to enhancing data security and encouraging greater data sharing and utilization.

Furthermore, the study underscores the importance of employee involvement and communication in mitigating resistance to organizational change. Actively involving healthcare professionals in decision-making and fostering open communication channels creates a sense of ownership and commitment to organizational goals. Moreover, the study highlights the role of corporate culture in influencing employee resistance to change. A positive and adaptable culture that embraces innovation and continuous improvement can foster positive attitudes toward change and innovation.

The implications of this study hold significant relevance for the healthcare industry. By addressing the identified challenges and implementing the proposed strategies, healthcare organizations can optimize E-Health system utilization, improving patient care experiences and organizational effectiveness. E-Health systems' successful adoption and utilization require a multifaceted approach and collaborative efforts among healthcare providers, administrators, and other stakeholders to embrace change and overcome barriers.

This study emphasizes the importance of fully embracing and effectively utilizing E-Health systems in healthcare practices. Healthcare organizations can optimize E-Health services, improve patient care outcomes, and enhance organizational efficiency by addressing barriers to change and underutilization. The practical recommendations and insights in this study offer valuable guidance for healthcare leaders seeking to maximize the potential of E-Health systems and deliver high-quality, patient-centered care. Through ongoing efforts and a commitment to innovation, the healthcare industry can harness the transformative power of E-Health systems to drive positive and sustainable outcomes for patients and organizations.

REFERENCES

Abuwarda, Z., Mostafa, K., Oetomo, A., Hegazy, T., & Morita, P. (2022). Wearable devices: Cross benefits from healthcare to construction. *Automation in Construction, 142*, 104501.

Acharya, P., Koirala, S., & Shrestha, A. (2019). Sampling techniques and sample size determination in research: A review. *Journal of Biomedical Sciences, 6, 1-7*. https://www.ncbi.nlm.nih.gov/pmc/articles/PMC6577056/

Akinyode, B. F., & Khan, T. H. (2018). Step by step approach for qualitative data analysis. *International Journal of built environment and sustainability, 5*(3). http://orcid.org/0000-0003-0578-2905

Alazzam, M. B., Al Khatib, H., Mohammad, W. T., & Alassery, F. (2021). E-healthE-Health system characteristics, medical performance, and healthcare quality at Jordan's health centers. *Journal of healthcare engineering, 2021*.

Albahri, O. S., Zaidan, A. A., Zaidan, B. B., Hashim, M., Albahri, A. S., & Alsalem, M. A. (2018). Real-time remote healthE-Health-monitoring Systems in a Medical Centre: A review of the provision of healthcare services-based body sensor information, open challenges and methodological aspects. *Journal of medical systems, 42*, 1-47.

Alexandru, A., & Ianculescu, M. (2019). Personalized Home HealthE-Healthcare Options for Smart Service Delivery and Patient-Centered Monitoring. *Journal of e-healthE-Health Management*.

Alhassan, A., Alshammari, N., Aljohani, N., & Mohammad, S. (2017). Factors influencing the adoption of mobile health apps for chronic disease management: A systematic review. Journal of Medical Internet Research, 19(7), e270. doi: https://10.2196/jmir.7458

Alpert, J. M., Dyer, K. E., & Lafata, J. E. (2017). Patient-centered communication in digital medical encounters. *Patient education and counseling*, *100*(10), 1852-1858.

Al-Radaideh, A. T., & Alazzam, M. (2020). Critical successful factors affecting the adoption of E-healthE-Health systems in developing countries. *Available at SSRN 3522884*.

Ames, H., Glenton, C., & Lewin, S. (2019). Purposive sampling in a qualitative evidence synthesis: A worked example from a synthesis on parental perceptions of vaccination communication. *Bmc medical research methodology*, *19*(1), 1–9. https://bmcmedresmethodol.biomedcentral.com/articles/10.1186/s12874-019-0665-4

Ammenwerth, E., Hoerbst, A., Lannig, S., Mueller, G., Siebert, U., & Schnell-Inderst, P. (2019). Effects of adult patient portals on patient empowerment and health-related outcomes: a systematic review. *MEDINFO 2019: Health and Wellbeing e-Networks for All*, 1106-1110. https://10.3233/SHTI190397

Andersen, T. O., Bansler, J. P., Kensing, F., Moll, J., Mønsted, T., Nielsen, K. D., Nielsen, O. W., Petersen, H. H., & Svendsen, J. H. (2018). Aligning Concerns in Telecare: Three Concepts to Guide the Design of Patient-Centred E-Health. *Computer Supported Cooperative Work (CSCW)*, *27*(3-6), 1181–1214. https://doi.org/10.1007/s10606-018-9309-1

Anshari, M., Almunawar, M. N., Younis, M. Z., & Kisa, A. (2021). Modeling users' empowerment in e-health systems. *Sustainability*, *13*(23), 12993.

Atasoy, H., Greenwood, B. N., & McCullough, J. S. (2019). The digitization of patient care: a review of the effects of electronic health records on health care quality and
utilization. *Annual review of public health*, *40*, 487-500. https://doi.org/10.1146/annurev-publhealth-040218-044206

Barbosa, S. D. F. F., & Dal Sasso, G. T. (2022). Patient Safety: Opportunities and Risks of Health IT Applications, Methods, and Devices. In *Nursing Informatics: A Health Informatics, Interprofessional and Global Perspective* (pp. 357-374). Cham: Springer International Publishing.

Bauer, G. (2018). Delivering value-based care with e-healthE-Health services. *Journal of healthcare management*, *63*(4), 251-260.

Baumann, L. A., Baker, J., & Elshaug, A. G. (2018). The impact of electronic health record systems on clinical documentation times: A systematic review. *Health policy*, *122*(8), 827-836. https://doi.org/10.1016/j.healthpol.2018.05.014

Bearman, M. (2019). Focus on methodology: Eliciting rich data: A practical approach to writing semi-structured interview schedules. *Focus on Health Professional Education: A Multi-Professional Journal*, *20*(3), 1-11. https://doi.org/10.11157/fohpe.v20i3.387

Biancone, P., Secinaro, S., Marseglia, R., & Calandra, D. (2021). E-healthE-Health for the future. Managerial perspectives using a multiple case study approach. *Technovation*, 102406.

Bou-Karroum, L., El-Harakeh, A., Kassamany, I., Ismail, H., El Arnaout, N., Charide, R., Madi, F., Jamali, S., Martineau, T., El-Jardali, F., & Akl, E. A. (2020). Health care workers in conflict and post-conflict settings: Systematic mapping of the evidence. *PLoS ONE, 15*(5). https://doi.org/10.1371/journal.pone.0233757

Calvillo-Arbizu, J., Roa-Romero, L. M., Estudillo-Valderrama, M. A., Salgueira-Lazo, M., Aresté-Fosalba, N., del-Castillo-Rodríguez, N. L., González-Cabrera, F., Marrero-

Robayna, S., López-de-la-Manzana, V., & Román-Martínez, I. (2019). User-centred design for developing e-Health system for renal patients at home (AppNephro).

International Journal of Medical Informatics, 125, 47–54. https://doi.org/10.1016/j.ijmedinf.2019.02.007

Campbell, S., Greenwood, M., Prior, S., Shearer, T., Walkem, K., Young, S., Bywaters, D., & Walker, K. (2020). Purposive Sampling: Complex or Simple? Research Case Examples. *Journal of Research in Nursing, 25*(8), 652–661. NCBI. https://doi.org/10.1177/1744987120927206

Castleberry, A., & Nolen, A. (2018). Thematic analysis of qualitative research data: Is it as easy as it sounds? *Currents in pharmacy teaching and learning, 10*(6), 807-815.

Collins, C. S., & Stockton, C. M. (2018). The central role of theory in qualitative research. *International journal of qualitative methods, 17*(1), 1609406918797475.

Coughlin, S., Prochaska, J., Williams, L. B., Besenyi, G., Heboyan, V., Goggans, S., Yoo, W., & De Leo, G. (2017). Patient web portals, disease management, and primary prevention.

Risk Management and Healthcare Policy, Volume 10, 33–40. https://doi.org/10.2147/rmhp.s130431

Coventry, L., & Branley, D. (2018). Cybersecurity in healthcare: A narrative review of trends, threats and ways forward. *Maturitas, 113,* 48-52.

Cypress, B. (2018). Qualitative research methods: A phenomenological focus. *Dimensions of Critical Care Nursing, 37*(6), 302-309. *DOI:* 10.1097

Dash, S., Shakyawar, S. K., Sharma, M., & Kaushik, S. (2019). Big data in healthcare: management, analysis and future prospects. *Journal of big data, 6*(1), 1-25. https://link.springer.com/article/10.1186/s40537-019-0217-0

Davis, F. D. (1989). Technology acceptance model: TAM. *Al-Suqri, MN, Al-Aufi, AS: Information Seeking Behavior and*

Technology Adoption, 205-219. https://quod.lib.umich.edu/b/busadwp/images/b/1/4/b1409190.0001.001.pdf

De Grood, C., Raissi, A., Kwon, Y., & Santana, M. J. (2016). Adoption of e-health technology by physicians: a scoping review. *Journal of multidisciplinary healthcare*, 335-344.

DeJonckheere, M., & Vaughn, L. M. (2019). Semistructured interviewing in primary care research: a balance of relationship and rigour. *Family medicine and community health*, 7(2). https://doi.org/10.1136%2Ffmch-2018-000057

Duggal, M., El Ayadi, A., Duggal, B., Reynolds, N., & Bascaran, C. (2023). Editorial: Challenges in implementing digital health in public health settings in low and middle income countries. Frontiers in public health, 10, 1090303. https://doi.org/10.3389/fpubh.2022.1090303

Dymyt, M. (2020). The Role of eHealth in the Management of Patient Safety. *Journal of e- healthE-Health Management, 2020*, 1-13.

Dymyt, M., & Dymyt, T. (2018). E-HEALTHE-HEALTH as a Tool for Strengthening the Role of a Patient in the Process of Providing Health Services. *MODERN/ MANAGEMENT/*, 21.

Errida, A., & Lotfi, B. (2021). The determinants of organizational change management success: Literature review and case study. *International Journal of Engineering Business Management, 13*, 18479790211016273.

Gerring, J. (2017). Qualitative methods. *Annual review of political science, 20*, 15-36. https://doi.org/10.1146/annurev-polisci-092415-024158

Glaser, B. G., & Strauss, A. L. (1968). The Discovery of Grounded Theory: Strategies for Qualitative Research.

Haleem, A., Javaid, M., Singh, R. P., & Suman, R. (2021). Telemedicine for healthcare: Capabilities, features, barriers, and applications. *Sensors International, 2*, 100117.

Iqbal, S., Kiah, M. L. M., Zaidan, A. A., Zaidan, B. B.,

Albahri, O. S., Albahri, A. S., & Alsalem, M. A. (2019). Real-time-based E-healthE-Health systems: Design and implementation of a lightweight key management protocol for securing sensitive information of patients. *Health and Technology*, *9*, 93-111.

Iyanna, S., Kaur, P., Ractham, P., Talwar, S., & Islam, A. N. (2022). Digital transformation of the healthE-Healthcare sector. What is impeding the adoption and continued usage of technology-driven innovations by end users? *Journal of Business Research*, *153*, 150- 161.

Johnson, W. G., Gee, P. M., Kelly, L. A., & Butler, R. J. (2021). The Effect of Electronic Medical Records on Nurses' Job Satisfaction: A Multi-Year Analysis. *Urban Studies and Public Administration, 4*(3), p1. https://doi.org/10.22158/uspa.v4n3p1

Kataria, S., & Ravindran, V. (2020). Electronic health records: a critical appraisal of strengths and limitations. *Journal of the Royal College of Physicians of Edinburgh*, *50*(3), 262-268.

Kegler, M. C., Raskind, I. G., Comeau, D. L., Griffith, D. M., Cooper, H. L., & Shelton, R. C. (2019). Study design and use of inquiry frameworks in qualitative research published in health education & behavior. *Health Education & Behavior*, *46*(1), 24–31. https://journals.sagepub.com/doi/abs/10.1177/1090198118795018

Kelly, J. T., Campbell, K. L., Gong, E., & Scuffham, P. (2020). The Internet of Things: Impact and implications for health care delivery. *Journal of medical Internet research*, *22*(11), e20135.

Kiger, M. E., & Varpio, L. (2020). Thematic analysis of qualitative data: AMEE Guide No. 131. *Medical teacher*, *42*(8), 846-854. https://doi.org/10.1080/0142159X.2020.1755030

Kim, J., & Lee, J. (2021). The role of e-health systems in enhancing client tracking in hospitals.

Healthcare Informatics Research, 27(4), 398-407. <u>https://</u>

www.clinicalleader.com/doc/the-role-of-e-health-technologies-in-clinical-care-and-research-0001

Kivekäs, E., Mikkonen, S., Borycki, E., Ihantola, S., & Saranto, K. (2018). Physicians' Estimates of Electronic Prescribing's Impact on Patient Safety and Quality of Care. *ACI Open*, 2(01), e30-e40. https://10.1055/s-0038-1660464

Knechel, N. (2019). What is in a sample? Why selecting the right research participants matters. *Journal of Emergency Nursing*, 45(3), 332–334. https://www.intljourtranur.com/article/S0099-1767(19)30041-8/abstract

Kruse, C. S., Stein, A., Thomas, H., & Kaur, H. (2018). The use of electronic health records to support population health: a systematic review of the literature. *Journal of medical systems*, 42, 1-16. https://doi.org/10.1007/s10916-018-1075-6

Lakens, D. (2022). Sample size justification. *Collabra: Psychology*, 8(1), 33267. Lamprinos, I. E. (2019). Novel e-Health and m-Health Services. In *Health Monitoring Systems* (pp. 227-242). CRC Press.

Laukka, E., Huhtakangas, M., Heponiemi, T., Kujala, S., Kaihlanen, A. M., Gluschkoff, K., & Kanste, O. (2020). Health care professionals' experiences of patient-professional communication over patient portals: systematic review of qualitative studies. *Journal of Medical Internet Research*, 22(12), e21623. https://doi.org/10.2196/21623

Liu, W., Zhu, S. S., Mundie, T., & Krieger, U. (2017, October). Advanced blockchain architecture for e-healthE-Health systems. In *2017 IEEE 19th International Conference on e-HealthE-Health Networking, Applications, and Services (Healthcom)* (pp. 1-6). IEEE.

Lokken, T. G., Blegen, R. N., Hoff, M. D., & Demaerschalk, B. M. (2020). Overview for implementation of telemedicine services in a large integrated multispecialty health care system. *Telemedicine and e-HealthE-Health*, 26(4), 382-387.

Maksimović, M., & Vujović, V. (2017). Internet of things based e-healthE-Health systems: ideas, expectations, and concerns. *Handbook of large-scale distributed computing in smart healthcare*, 241-280.

Manzini, F., Diehl, E. E., Farias, M. R., dos Santos, R. I., Soares, L., Rech, N., Lorenzoni, A. A., & Leite, S. N. (2020). Analysis of a Blended, In-Service, Continuing Education Course in a Public Health System: Lessons for Education Providers and Healthcare Managers.

Frontiers in Public Health, 8. https://doi.org/10.3389/fpubh. 2020.561238

Massoudi, B., Holvast, F., Bockting, C. L., Burger, H., & Blanker, M. H. (2019). The effectiveness and cost-effectiveness of e-healthE-Health interventions for depression and anxiety in primary care: A systematic review and meta-analysis. *Journal of affective disorders, 245*, 728-743.

McGraw, D., & Mandl, K. D. (2021). Privacy protections to encourage use of health-relevant digital data in a learning health system. *NPJ digital medicine, 4*(1), 2.

Miah, S. J., Hasan, J., & Gammack, J. G. (2017). On-cloud healthcare clinic: an E-Health consultancy approach for remote communities in a developing country. *Telematics and Informatics, 34*(1), 311-322.

Mickan, S. M., Tilson, J. K., Atherton, H., Roberts, N. W., & Heneghan, C. J. (2019). Evidence of effectiveness of health care professionals using handheld computers: a scoping review of systematic reviews. *Journal of Medical Internet Research, 21*(10), e13128. Doi: 10.2196/13128 https://www.jmir.org/2019/10/e13128/

Mishra, P., Pandey, C. M., Singh, U., Gupta, A., Sahu, C., & Keshri, A. (2019). Descriptive statistics and normality tests for statistical data. *Annals of cardiac anaesthesia, 22*(1), 67.

Mitnik, P. A. (2020). Intergenerational Income Elasticities, Instrumental Variable Estimation, and Bracketing Strategies. *Sociological Methodology, 50*(1), 1–46. https://doi.org/10.1177/0081175019887992

Mohajan, H. K. (2018). Qualitative research methodology in

social sciences and related subjects. *Journal of economic development, environment, and People, 7*(1), 23-48. https://www.ceeol.com/search/article-detail?id=640546

Moloney, W., Fieldes, J., & Jacobs, S. (2020). An integrative review of how healthcare organizations can support hospital nurses to thrive at work. *International journal of environmental research and public health, 17*(23), 8757.

Moon, M. D. (2019). Triangulation: A method to increase validity, reliability, and legitimation in clinical research. *Journal of emergency nursing, 45*(1), 103-105.

Mshali, H., Lemlouma, T., Moloney, M., & Magoni, D. (2018). A survey on health monitoring systems for health smart homes. *International Journal of Industrial Ergonomics, 66,* 26- 56.

Nguyen, M., Fujioka, J., Wentlandt, K., Onabajo, N., Wong, I., Bhatia, R. S., Bhattacharyya, O., & Stamenova, V. (2020). Using the technology acceptance model to explore health provider and administrator perceptions of the usefulness and ease of using technology in palliative care. *BMC Palliative Care, 19*(1). https://doi.org/10.1186/s12904-020-00644-8

Potnuru, R. K. G., Sharma, R., & Sahoo, C. K. (2023). Employee voice, employee involvement, and organizational change readiness: mediating role of commitment-to-change and moderating role of transformational leadership. *Business Perspectives and Research, 11*(3), 355-371. https://doi.org/10.1177/22785337211043962

Prabhu, G. N. (2020). Teaching the scope and limits of generalizability in qualitative research. *New Trends in Qualitative Research, 1,* 186-192.

Qandeel, M. S. (2022). *A systematic literature review: choice bracketing in decision making.* https://www.researchsquare.com/article/rs-2304198/latest.pdf

Raj, C., Jain, C., & Arif, W. (2017, March). HEMAN: Health monitoring and nous: An IoT- based e-healthE-Health care system for remote telemedicine. In *2017 International conference on wireless communications, signal processing and networking (WiSPNET)* (pp. 2115-2119). IEEE

Ratwani, R. M. (2017). Electronic health records and improved patient care: opportunities for applied psychology. *Current directions in psychological science*, *26*(4), 359-365. https://doi.org/10.1177/0963721417700691

Richards, K. A. R., & Hemphill, M. A. (2018). A practical guide to collaborative qualitative data analysis. *Journal of Teaching in Physical education*, *37*(2), 225-231. https://doi.org/ 10.1123/jtpe.2017-0084

Risling, T., Martinez, J., Young, J., & Thorp-Froslie, N. (2017). Evaluating patient empowerment in association with eHealth technology: scoping review. *Journal of medical Internet research*, *19*(9), e329. https://doi.org/10.2196/jmir.7809

Roulston, K., & Choi, M. (2018). Qualitative interviews. *The SAGE handbook of qualitative data collection*, 233-249. http://digital.casalini.it/9781526416063

Santana, R. F., Pereira, S. K., do Carmo, T. G., Freire, V. E. C. D. S., Soares, T. D. S., do Amaral, D. M., & Vaqueiro, R. D. (2018). Effectiveness of a telephone follow- up nursing inter-vention in postsurgical patients. *International Journal of Nursing Practice*, *24*(4), e12648.

Sharikh, E. A., Shannak, R., Suifan, T., & Ayaad, O. (2020). The impact of electronic medical records' functions on the quality of health services. *British Journal of Healthcare Management*, *26*(2), 1-13. https://doi.org/10.12968/bjhc. 2019.0056

Sivan, R., & Zukarnain, Z. A. (2021). Security and privacy in cloud-based e-health system. *Symmetry*, *13*(5), 742. https:// doi.org/10.3390/sym13050742

Sneha, S., & Straub, D. (2017). E-Health: Value proposition and technologies enabling collaborative Healthcare. http://hdl. handle.net/10125/41260

Stoll, C. R., Izadi, S., Fowler, S., Green, P., Suls, J., & Colditz, G. A. (2019). The value of a second reviewer for study selection in systematic reviews. *Research Synthesis Methods*, *10*(4), 539-545. https://onlinelibrary.wiley.com/doi/abs/10.1002/jrsm.1369

Sullivan, A. L., Sadeh, S., & Houri, A. K. (2019). Are school psychologists' special education eligibility decisions reliable and unbiased: A multi-study experimental investigation. *Journal of school psychology*, pp. *77*, 90–109. https://www.sciencedirect.com/science/article/pii/S0022440519300895

Susanto, H., & Chen, C. K. (2017). Information and communication emerging technology: making sense of healthcare innovation. *Internet of things and big data technologies for next generation healthcare*, 229-250.

Taherdoost, H. (2018). A review of technology acceptance and adoption models and theories. *Procedia manufacturing*, *22*, 960-967.

Tebeje, T. H., & Klein, J. (2021). Applications of e-health to support person-centered health care at the time of COVID-19 pandemic. *Telemedicine and e-Health*, *27*(2), 150-158. https://doi.org/10.1089/tmj.2020.0201

Thomas, D. R. (2016). Feedback from research participants: are member checks useful in qualitative research? *Qualitative research in psychology*, *14*(1), 23-41.

Thomas, L. B., Mastorides, S. M., Viswanadhan, N. A., Jakey, C. E., & Borkowski, A. A. (2021). Artificial intelligence: review of current and future applications in medicine. *Federal Practitioner*, *38*(11), 527. https://doi.org/10.12788/fp.0174

Tremoulet, P. D., Regli, S. H., & Krishnan, R. (2020). Design for effective care collaboration.

In *Design for Health* (pp. 103-125). Academic Press. https://doi.org/10.1016/B978-0-12-816427-3.00006-3

Tubaishat, A. (2017). Perceived usefulness and perceived ease of use of electronic health records among nurses: Application of Technology Acceptance Model. *Informatics for Health and Social Care*, *43*(4), 379-389. https://doi.org/10.1080/17538157.2017.1363761

Wahyuni, R. (2017). Explaining acceptance of e-health services: An extension of TAM and health belief model approach. In *2017 5th International Conference on Cyber and IT Service Management (CITSM)* (pp. 1-7). IEEE.

Wang, C., Wu, X., & Qi, H. (2021, December). A comprehensive analysis of e-health literacy research focuses and trends. In *Healthcare* (Vol. 10, No. 1, p. 66). MDPI.

Wu, V. X., Dong, Y., Tan, P. C., Gan, P., Zhang, D., Chi, Y., Chao, F. F. T., Lu, J., Teo, B. H.D., & Tan, Y. Q. (2022). Development of a Community-Based e-Health Program for Older Adults With Chronic Diseases: Pilot Pre-Post Study. *JMIR Aging, 5*(1), e33118. https://doi.org/10.2196/33118

Xu, H., Granger, B. B., Drake, C. D., Peterson, E. D., & Dupre, M. E. (2022). Effectiveness of telemedicine visits in reducing 30- day readmissions among patients with heart failure during the COVID- 19 pandemic. *Journal of the American Heart Association, 11*(7),e023935. https://doi.org/10.1161/JAHA.121.023935

Yusif, S., Hafeez-Baig, A., & Soar, J. (2017). e-Health readiness assessment factors and measuring tools: A systematic review. *International journal of medical informatics, 107*, 56-64.

Zhang, J., Dushaj, K., Rasquinha, V. J., Scuderi, G. R., & Hepinstall, M. S. (2019). Monitoring surgical incision sites in orthopedic patients using an online physician-patient messaging platform. *The Journal of arthroplasty, 34*(9), 1897-1900.

LETTER TO THE FACILITY REQUESTING ACCESS PERMISSION (APPENDIX A)

Name:

Date: /   /

Management Golden Years Care Facility
Address: 108 Woodward Rd, Manalapan,
NJ 07726

RE: Request an appointment date to access the facility and interview experienced employees regarding the E-Health system.

I kindly request permission to access the facility on the date........................ for five-hour from 8 a.m. to 1 p.m. I will interview participants who have experience using the E-Health system. The data collected will help me complete my research successfully and might also be helpful to the facility by identifying areas for improvement.

Yours Sincerely

Signature

LIST OF INTERVIEW QUESTIONS (APPENDIX B)

1. How has implementing the E-Health system impacted the workflow and efficiency of healthcare delivery at Golden Years Care facility?
2. What are the main benefits and drawbacks of E-Health systems in improving patient care and outcomes at Golden Years Care facility?
3. How have the staff members adapted to the E-Health system, and what challenges have they encountered during the implementation process?
4. How have patients responded to and experienced using the E-Health system in their care at Golden Years Care facility?
5. In what ways has the E-Health system changed communication and collaboration between healthcare providers at Golden Years Care facility?
6. What role does the E-Health system play in facilitating remote monitoring and telemedicine services at Golden Years Care facility?
7. How are the security and privacy of patient data ensured when using the E-Health system at Golden Years Care facility?
8. What specific challenges or difficulties have you Observed when using the E-Health system at Golden Years Care facility?